Advances and Controversies in Hematopoietic Transplantation and Cell Therapy

Series Editors
Syed A. Abutalib
Deerfield, Illinois, USA

James O. Armitage
Omaha, Nebraska, USA

Each volume will focus on different aspects of blood and marrow transplantation or cellular therapy and presents up-to-date data and concepts as well as controversial aspects.

More information about this series at http://www.springer.com/series/13907

Joseph Schwartz • Beth H. Shaz
Editors

Best Practices in Processing and Storage for Hematopoietic Cell Transplantation

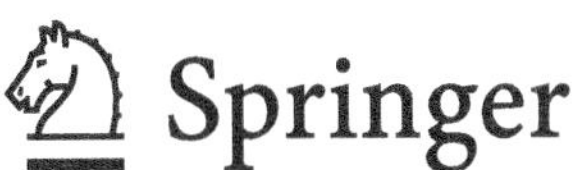

Editors
Joseph Schwartz
Department of Pathology & Cell Biology
Columbia University
New York, NY
USA

Beth H. Shaz
New York Blood Center
New York, NY
USA

Advances and Controversies in Hematopoietic Transplantation and Cell Therapy
ISBN 978-3-319-86517-1 ISBN 978-3-319-58949-7 (eBook)
https://doi.org/10.1007/978-3-319-58949-7

Printed on acid-free paper

This Springer imprint is published by Springer Nature
The registered company is Springer International Publishing AG
The registered company address is: Gewerbestrasse 11, 6330 Cham, Switzerland

Contents

Journey of Hematopoietic Cells: Processing to Infusion

1

Beth Shaz and Joseph Schwartz

1.1 Introduction

Hematopoietic cell transplantation (HCT) is a lifesaving therapy. Almost 20,000 transplants were performed in the United States in 2014. Transplantation is used to treat a wide variety of diseases, most commonly leukemias, lymphomas, multiple myeloma, and certain solid tumors. More recently, its use had been expanded to nonmalignant disorders, such as thalassemia and sickle cell disease. HCT sources include bone marrow, peripheral blood, and cord blood. To maintain a high-quality product to ensure engraftment and optimal patient outcomes, each step of the process must be performed appropriately, including donor qualification, collection, processing, storage and transportation, and infusion. Transplantation logistics and care are overseen by accrediting and regulatory agencies (see Chap. 2). Data from the United States are tracked through HRSA (Health Resources and Services Administration) and CIBMTR (Center for International Blood and Marrow Transplant Research) (Center for International Blood & Marrow Transplant Research 2017). The field continues to improve patient outcomes and expand clinical indications as new processing techniques and medications become available.

B. Shaz, M.D. (✉)
New York Blood Center, New York, NY, USA

Department of Pathology and Cell Biology,
College of Physician and Surgeons of Columbia University, New York, NY, USA
e-mail: bshaz@nybc.org

J. Schwartz, M.D.
Department of Pathology and Cell Biology, College of Physician and Surgeons of Columbia University, New York, NY, USA

Transfusion Medicine & Cellular Therapy Service, Columbia University Medical Center Campus, New York Presbyterian Hospital, New York, NY, USA

J. Schwartz, B.H. Shaz (eds.), *Best Practices in Processing and Storage for Hematopoietic Cell Transplantation*, Advances and Controversies in Hematopoietic Transplantation and Cell Therapy,
https://doi.org/10.1007/978-3-319-58949-7_1

1.2 The Basic Tenets of Donor Eligibility

Assessing hematopoietic graft donors for eligibility protects both the donor and the recipient. Each graft source has different recipient risk and different patient outcomes. The source may be chosen based on recipient need or donor availability. Peripheral blood is the source of graft in 84% of the US transplants and almost all of the autologous transplants (Center for International Blood & Marrow Transplant Research 2017). Cord blood is mostly used for unrelated transplants, while bone marrow and peripheral blood are used similarly in related and unrelated transplants. Cord blood is collected, cryopreserved, and stored awaiting patient need, while peripheral blood and bone marrow are collected for a specific patient. Thus cord blood units can be obtained more quickly than other sources. However cord blood units have a fixed cell dose; thus without enhancement, such as expanding cells or supplying another manipulated or unmanipulated unit, they are limited to be used in smaller (defined by body weight) recipients (see Chaps. 8 and 9). Cord blood is the lowest risk to the donor, followed by peripheral blood as the donor needs to be stimulated by G-CSF and undergoes a long apheresis procedure, and lastly bone marrow as the donor usually undergoes anesthesia and long volume collection. For all donors, infectious disease screening is performed, and informed consent is obtained (in the case of cord blood from the mother). Eligibility criteria and donor testing are regulated through the FDA, FACT, AABB, as well as other organizations (see Chap. 3).

1.3 The Basic Tenets of Collection

Each hematopoietic progenitor cell (HPC) product is collected differently depending on the graft source. Cord blood products (HPC, cord blood) are collected from the cord blood when the placenta is still in utero or after delivery. The goal is to obtain the highest number of total nucleated cells (TNCs)/kg of recipient body weight. $CD34^+$ cells from peripheral blood (HPC, apheresis) are collected by apheresis after a donor is stimulated with G-CSF for a minimum of 5 days. For autologous donors sometimes $CD34^+$ cell mobilization takes longer, or an alternate agent, plerixafor (CXCR4 antagonist), is also needed. The desired collected cell dose depends on the weight of the recipient, usually $\geq 2 \times 10^6$ $CD34^+$ cells/kg of recipient body weight. The $CD34^+$ cell dose in the HPC, apheresis is usually higher than other products. Most healthy allogeneic donors can undergo apheresis through peripheral access, although some autologous and allogenic donors may need to have central line placed. The apheresis procedure can be long as multiple total blood volumes (TBVs) are processed in a single collection. Bone marrow (HPC, bone marrow) is harvested from the iliac crest through multiple aspirations in an operating room. The desired collected cell dose depends on the weight of the recipient, usually $\geq 3 \times 10^8$ TNC/kg of recipient body weight or 10–15 ml of bone marrow/kg of recipient body weight. For all units once collected they are sent to a processing facility prior to infusion.

1.4 The Basic Tenets of Processing and Storage

Products are transferred at room temperature or at 2–8 °C from collection to processing facility, depending on the product and time of transportation. Processing depends on the graft source, ABO compatibility between donor and recipient, and need for cryopreservation. If there is major ABO incompatibility, recipient has antibodies to donor RBCs, and then RBCs may need to be removed from the product. Since most HPC, apheresis products have low RBC volume, they typically are not RBC reduced. HPC, bone marrow products have high hematocrits and RBC volume so RBCs would be removed. Some cord blood banks remove RBCs from all products because during cryopreservation RBCs lyse. If there is minor ABO incompatibility, donor plasma has antibodies to recipient RBCs, then plasma is removed from the product, termed plasma reduction, from HPC, apheresis and HPC, bone marrow. Plasma is typically removed during cord blood processing. If both major and minor incompatiblity exists (termed bidrectional ABO incompatibility), RBCs and plasma may need to be removed from the product.

Other HPC product processing includes cell selection, either enriching for CD34$^+$ cells or depleting T cells, with an aim to mitigate graft-versus-host disease.

If products are not infused shortly, typically within 72 h, after collection then they are cryopreserved. Most cell processing laboratories cryopreserve grafts in dimethyl sulfoxide (DMSO) and source of plasma protein. DMSO prevents cellular dehydration and ice crystal formation in the cells (Shaz et al. 2013). The product is immediately frozen once DMSO is added, either at a controlled or uncontrolled rate freezing. Products are then typically stored in the *vapor phase* of liquid nitrogen, <−150 °C. All cord blood units are cryopreserved and stored in a cord blood bank for future use. Autologous HPCs are cryopreserved until the donor/recipient has undergone preparative regimens. Most allogenic bone marrow and apheresis HPCs are infused fresh.

1.5 The Basic Tenets of Distribution and Infusion

HPC products are then distributed to the infusing facility. Cryopreserved products are typically shipped to facilities in a dry shipper to maintain temperatures. Cryopreserved products are then thawed at 37 °C at the patient's bedside and infused immediately. A filter to remove cellular debris, but not a leukoreduction filter, can be used. DMSO can be removed through washing to mitigate most adverse events in selected situations (see Chaps. 7 and 11). However, such washing results in cell loss. No more than 1 g DMSO/kg of recipient weight should be infused daily.

1.6 Expert Point of View

Patient outcome depends on high-quality process from donor selection to infusion. Each step of the process requires validation and quality control. Bone marrow, apheresis, and cord blood HPCs have an important role in HCT, and patient access to all three enables tailoring treatments to patients' needs and product availability. Although each cellular processing laboratory acts as individuals, the overall tenets of collection, processing, storage, distribution, and infusion are similar.

1.7 Future Directions

The emergence of HLA-haploidentical transplants has resulted changes in HPC processing, such as cell selection. To improve engraftment times after cord blood transplantation, cell expansion or engraftment-enhancing technologies are being explored. The early success of immunotherapy may change the use of HCT. All of these changes result in improved patient outcomes.

References

Center for International Blood & Marrow Transplant Research (2017) www.cibmtr.org. Accessed 23 March 2017

Health Resources and Services Administration (2017) Bone marrow and cord blood donation and transplantation. https://bloodcell.transplant.hrsa.gov/. Accessed 23 March 2017

Shaz BH, Hillyer CD, Mikhail R, Abrams CS (eds) (2013) Transfusion medicine and hemostasis: clinical and laboratory aspects, 2nd edn. Elsevier, Oxford, UK

Regulations and Accreditation of Processing Laboratories

2

Yvette C. Tanhehco and Joseph Schwartz

2.1 Introduction

Cellular therapy products are highly regulated in the United States both at the state and federal levels. The Food and Drug Administration (FDA) and Centers for Medicare and Medicaid Services (CMS) are the main governing bodies that provide federal oversight. State health departments may also have local regulations for processing laboratories. Individuals and organizations or institutions involved in cellular therapy processing must be familiar with the requirements of these agencies (Table 2.1).

Table 2.1 Federal agencies with regulations for processing laboratories

Regulatory agency	Abbreviation
Food and Drug Administration	FDA
Center for Medicaid and Medicare Services	CMS
Environmental Protection Agency	EPA
Occupational Safety and Health Administration	OSHA
Local State Department of Health	Local state DOH

Y.C. Tanhehco, Ph.D., M.D., M.S. (✉)
Transfusion Medicine and Cellular Therapy, NewYork-Presbyterian Hospital, New York, NY, USA

Hemotherapy and Cellular Therapy, NewYork-Presbyterian Hospital, New York, NY, USA

Department of Pathology and Cell Biology, Columbia University, New York, NY, USA
e-mail: yct2103@cumc.columbia.edu

J. Schwartz, M.D., M.P.H.
Transfusion Medicine and Cellular Therapy, NewYork-Presbyterian Hospital, New York, NY, USA

Department of Pathology and Cell Biology, Columbia University, New York, NY, USA

J. Schwartz, B.H. Shaz (eds.), *Best Practices in Processing and Storage for Hematopoietic Cell Transplantation*, Advances and Controversies in Hematopoietic Transplantation and Cell Therapy,
https://doi.org/10.1007/978-3-319-58949-7_2

Table 2.2 Title 21 FDA regulations relevant to processing laboratories

Part	Topic
210	Current good manufacturing practice in manufacturing, processing, packing, or holding of drugs
211	Current good manufacturing practice for finished pharmaceuticals
1270	Human tissue intended for transplantation
Subpart A	General provisions
Subpart B	Donor screening and testing
Subpart C	Procedures and records
Subpart D	Inspection of tissue establishments
1271	Human cells, tissues, and cellular and tissue-based products
Subpart A	General provisions
Subpart B	Procedures for registration and listing
Subpart C	Donor eligibility
Subpart D	Current good tissue practice
Subpart E	Additional requirements for establishments described in 1271.10
Subpart F	Inspection and enforcement of establishment described in 1271.10

Cellular therapy processing laboratories may also be accredited by organizations such as the FACT, JACIE, or AABB. While regulations have the force of law, accreditation standards are not legally binding. Accreditation allows an organization or institution to be officially recognized as being highly qualified to perform cellular therapy activities and to have a high quality of operations. The US federal government has granted deemed status to certain accreditation organizations that have standards and a survey process that meets or exceeds Medicare and Medicaid requirements. Laboratories that achieve accreditation through an organization's "deemed status" survey are determined to meet or exceed federal requirements. A list of accreditation organizations for processing laboratories is provided in Table 2.2.

2.2 U.S Food and Drug Administration

The general and permanent rules published in the Federal Register by the departments and agencies of the federal government are codified in the Code of Federal Regulations (CFR). The CFR includes 50 titles that represent broad areas subject to federal regulation. The 50 subject matter titles contain one or more individual volumes, which are updated once each calendar year, on a staggered basis. Titles 1–16 are revised as of January 1, titles 17–27 are revised as of April 1, titles 28–41 are revised as of July 1, and titles 42–50 are revised as of October 1 of each calendar year. Each title is further divided into chapters, which usually bear the name of the issuing agency. Each chapter is subdivided into parts that cover specific regulatory areas. Large parts may be subdivided into subparts. All parts are organized in sections, and most citations to the CFR refer to material at the section level (GPO n.d.).

FDA also publishes documents that represent the agency's current thinking on a certain topic. These guidance documents are non-binding nor do they create or confer any rights to individuals. Alternative approaches may be used to the one described in the guidance document if such approach satisfies the requirements of the applicable statute, regulations, or both (FDA n.d.).

Human cells or tissue intended for implantation, transplantation, infusion, or transfer into a human recipient is regulated as a human cell, tissue, and cellular and tissue-based product or HCT/P. Regulations relevant to cellular therapy processing laboratories are outlined in Table 2.2. The Center for Biologics Evaluation and Research (CBER) regulates HCT/Ps under 21 CFR Parts 1270 and 1271. Tissues regulated under these regulations include not only hematopoietic stem/progenitor cells derived from peripheral and cord blood but also the bone, skin, corneas, ligaments, tendons, dura mater, heart valves, oocytes, and semen. 21 Parts 1270 and 1271 require tissue establishments to screen and test donors, to prepare and follow written procedures for the prevention of the spread of communicable disease, and to maintain records (U.S. Food and Drug Administration n.d.-a).

FDA was granted authority to establish regulations for all HCT/Ps by Section 361 of the Public Health Service (PHS) Act. FDA requirements are aimed at protecting the public health by preventing the introduction, transmission, and spread of communicable disease while minimizing regulatory burden to tissue establishments. The three final rules published by FDA broaden the scope of products subject to regulation and include more comprehensive requirements. One final rule requires firms to register and list their HCT/Ps with FDA. The second rule requires tissue establishments to evaluate donors, through screening and testing, to reduce the transmission of infectious diseases through tissue transplantation. The third final rule establishes current good tissue practices for HCT/Ps. FDA's revised regulations are contained in Part 1271 and apply to tissues recovered after May 25, 2005 (U.S. Food and Drug Administration n.d.-a).

An HCT/P is regulated solely under Section 361 of the PHS Act and 21 CFR Part 1271 if it meets all of the following criteria (21 CFR 1271.10(a)) (U.S. Food and Drug Administration n.d.-b):

1. The HCT/P is minimally manipulated as defined below:
   (a) For structural tissue, processing that does not alter the original relevant characteristics of the tissue relating to the tissue's utility for reconstruction, repair, or replacement
   (b) For cells or nonstructural tissues, processing that does not alter the relevant biological characteristics of cells or tissues
2. The HCT/P is intended for homologous use only, as reflected by the labeling, advertising, or other indications of the manufacturer's objective intent.
3. The manufacture of the HCT/P does not involve the combination of the cells or tissues with another article, except for water, crystalloids, or a sterilizing, preserving, or storage agent, provided that the addition of water, crystalloids, or the sterilizing, preserving, or storage agent does not raise new clinical safety concerns with respect to the HCT/P.

4. Either:
   (a) The HCT/P does not have a systemic effect and is not dependent upon the metabolic activity of living cells for its primary function.
   (b) The HCT/P has a systemic effect or is dependent upon the metabolic activity of living cells for its primary function and:
      - Is for autologous use
      - Is for allogeneic use in a first-degree or second-degree blood relative
      - Is for reproductive use

If an HCT/P does not meet one or more of the criteria listed above, it will be regulated as a drug, device, and/or biological product under the Food, Drug, and Cosmetic Act (FD and C Act), and/or Section 351 (referred to as "351" HCT/Ps) of the PHS Act. Applicable regulations under 21 CFR Part 1271 and pre-market review will be required to obtain an FDA license. During the development phase, an investigational new drug (IND) or investigational device exemption (IDE) application must be submitted to the FDA before studies involving humans are initiated. Manufacturers of such HCT/Ps are required to comply with the regulations in 21 CFR Part 1271 and all the regulations for drugs, devices, or biological products, as applicable.

HCT/Ps derived from the peripheral blood or cord blood for use in a first- or second-degree blood relative or for autologous use that meet all the criteria in 21 CFR 1271.10(a) are regulated as "361" HCT/Ps. HCT/Ps derived from peripheral blood from unrelated donors are regulated as 351 products. These regulations remain under a period of delayed implementation for some clinical indications. Minimally manipulated, unrelated umbilical cord blood intended for hematopoietic or immunologic reconstitution in patients with disorders affecting the hematopoietic system must be FDA-licensed or used under an IND. Minimally manipulated bone marrow that is not combined with another regulated article (with some exceptions) and is intended for homologous use is not considered an HCT/P.

Manufacturers of HCT/P are required by FDA regulations in 21 CFR Part 1271 to have a tracking and labeling system that enables each product to be tracked from the donor to the recipient and from the recipient back to the donor. These manufacturers are also required to inform the facilities that receive the products of the tracking system that they have established. Facilities that only receive, store, and administer cells or tissues but do not perform any manufacturing steps are not subject to FDA's regulations regarding HCT/Ps, including the requirements for tracking. These activities are regulated by other standards such as The Joint Commission's (TJC) hospital standards for receipt, handling, and tracing of tissues as well as investigating adverse events.

FDA requires institutions that manufacture HCT/Ps to register with the agency and list their HCT/Ps. Manufacturing includes any steps involved in the recovery, processing, storage, labeling, packaging or distribution of HCT/Ps, and the screening or testing of the cell or tissue donor. Domestic and foreign establishments that manufacture, repack, or relabel drug and biologic products, including vaccines, are also required to register with the FDA and list all of their commercially marketed drug and biologic products. The FDA maintains a catalog of all drugs and biologics in commercial distribution in the United States (U.S. Food and Drug Administration n.d.-c). FDA also inspects laboratories that manufacture or process FDA-regulated products such as HCT/P processing laboratories, vaccine and drug manufacturers, and blood banks to verify that they comply with relevant regulations (U.S. Food and Drug Administration n.d.-d).

2.3 Center for Medicare and Medicaid Services

CMS regulates all US medical laboratories under the Clinical Laboratory Improvement Amendments (CLIA, 42 USC 263(a) and 42 CFR 493) to Section 353 of the Public Health Service Act. The objective of the CLIA program is to ensure quality laboratory testing (CMS n.d.-a). Regulations require that laboratories be certified under CLIA as both a general requirement and a prerequisite for receiving Medicare and Medicaid reimbursement. They provide minimal standards for facilities, equipment, and personnel (CMS n.d.-b). In order to be certified, laboratories must fulfill the following requirements:

1. Adequate facilities and equipment
2. Supervisory and technical personnel with training and experience appropriate to the complexity of testing
3. Quality management system
4. Successful ongoing performance in a CMS-approved proficiency testing (PT) program

All laboratories must register with CMS, submit to inspection by CMS or one of its "deemed status" partners, and obtain recertification every 2 years (Rauch 2007).

Laboratory tests are classified as waived tests or nonwaived tests according to their level of complexity. Waived tests are simple laboratory tests and procedures that require minimal training for the user. They pose an insignificant risk of erroneous results because they are so simple and accurate as to render the likelihood of erroneous results by the user negligible, and there is no unreasonable risk of harm to the patient if performed incorrectly (CDC n.d.-a). Waived tests include certain tests listed in the CLIA regulations, tests cleared by the FDA for home use, and tests approved for waiver by the FDA using the CLIA criteria. Laboratories that perform only waived tests register with CMS for a certificate of waiver. Some examples of waived tests include urine qualitative dipstick, nonautomated hemoglobin by copper sulfate, glucose monitoring devices, and spun hematocrit (U.S. Food and Drug Administration n.d.-e).

Nonwaived tests are further subcategorized as either moderate complexity or high complexity. Laboratories that perform these tests are required to have a CLIA certificate, submit to inspection, and meet the CLIA quality standards described in 42 CFR Subparts H, J, K, and M (CDC n.d.-b). FDA maintains a test complexity database that can be used to determine the complexity of a test system (U.S. Food and Drug Administration n.d.-f). Compatibility testing with manual reagents and infectious disease testing are examples of high complexity testing.

CLIA requires all laboratories performing even one test on "materials derived from the human body for the purpose of providing information for the diagnosis, prevention, or treatment of any disease or impairment of, or the assessment of the health of, human beings" to meet certain federal requirements. Laboratories performing tests for these purposes are considered under CLIA and must apply and obtain a certificate from the CLIA program that reflects the complexity of tests performed (CMS n.d.-c). Cellular therapy laboratories may obtain one of three types of certificates which is effective for 2 years: (1) certificate of compliance (State Department of Health conducts an inspection of laboratories performing nonwaived testing and determines that the laboratory is compliant with all applicable CLIA requirements), (2) certificate of accreditation (CMS-approved accreditation organization accredits laboratory that performs nonwaived testing), and (3) CMS-exempt status (licensure programs for nonwaived laboratories in New York and Washington States that are accepted by CMS) (CMS n.d.-c).

CMS has approved six laboratory accreditation organizations with requirements that meet CMS regulations: (1) the American Association of Blood Banks (AABB), (2) American Osteopathic Association (AOA), (3) American Society for Histocompatibility and Immunogenetics (ASHI), (4) College of American Pathologists (CAP), (5) former Commission on Office Laboratory Accreditation (COLA), and (6) The Joint Commission (CMS n.d.-d). The Joint Commission has cooperative agreements with ASHI, CAP, and COLA to accept their laboratory accreditations in facility surveys (The Joint Commission n.d.). CMS may perform its own follow-up surveys to validate those of the accreditation organizations.

CMS requires laboratories that hold certificates for nonwaived testing to participate and have satisfactory performance in a proficiency testing (PT) program. CMS regulations specify the tests and procedures (regulated analytes) that must pass approved PT if the laboratory performs them. A list of CLIA-approved proficiency testing providers can be found on the CMS website (CMS n.d.-e). CMS can revoke certification or impose fines on laboratories that fail to comply with its regulations.

2.4 Accreditation

Unlike regulations, accreditation is voluntary. The goal of accreditation is to verify compliance with standards and to assist in improving the quality of services provided. Accreditation informs patients, health insurance companies, and governments that your processing laboratory is dedicated to excellence and high-quality practices. Verification of compliance with standards is accomplished by peer review assessments. Several organizations (Table 2.3) provide accreditation for processing laboratories such as the Foundation for the Accreditation of Cellular Therapy (FACT), American Association of Blood Banks (AABB), and College of American Pathologists (CAP).

Table 2.3 Cellular therapy accreditation organizations

Accreditation organization	Abbreviation	Standards review cycle	Inspection frequency
American Association of Blood Banks	AABB	2 years	Every 2 years
College of American Pathologists	CAP	1 year	Every 2 years
Foundation for the Accreditation of Cellular Therapy	FACT	3 years	Every 3 years
Joint Accreditation Committee-ISBT and EBMT	JACIE	3 years	Every 4 years
National Marrow Donor Program	NMDP	2 years	N/A
World Marrow Donor Association	WMDA	5 years	Every 2 years (internal self-evaluation)
The Joint Commission	TJC	Ongoing	Every 36 months
Alliance for Harmonization of Cellular Therapy Accreditation	AHCTA	N/A	N/A

N/A not applicable

2.4.1 Foundation for the Accreditation of Cellular Therapy (FACT)

The Foundation for the Accreditation of Cellular Therapy (FACT) was cofounded in 1996 by the International Society for Cellular Therapy (ISCT) and the American Society of Blood and Marrow Transplantation (ASBMT) for the purposes of voluntary inspection and accreditation in the field of cellular therapy (U.S. Food and Drug Administration n.d.-b).

FACT Standards for hematopoietic progenitor cells (HPC), umbilical cord blood (UCB), and immune effector cells are developed by a committee of expert clinicians, scientists, technologists, and quality individuals. A new edition of the FACT Standards is published every 3 years. FACT Standards address the collection, processing, and administration of cellular therapies.

The accreditation process (Fig. 2.1) involves reviewing the current edition of the Standards and determining eligibility requirements. The eligibility application must be completed and submitted online. Initial applicants must submit a nonrefundable registration fee as well. Once the eligibility application is approved by FACT, the compliance application must be completed within 12 months to indicate compliance with the appropriate Standards. Each organization is assigned a FACT Accreditation Coordinator to assist with questions or concerns, request any additional or missing documentation, and communicate information between FACT and your organization such as the inspection date and inspection team. An on-site inspection will be conducted on one of the potential dates submitted by the organization. During the on-site inspection, the organization will provide a short overview of the program. The inspectors will visit all facilities and complete the inspection checklist. Compliance with the Standards is determined by evaluation of written documents provided by the organization and by a scheduled on-site inspection. At the end of the inspection, the inspectors will summarize their general impressions but will not make any accreditation determinations. The inspectors will submit an inspection

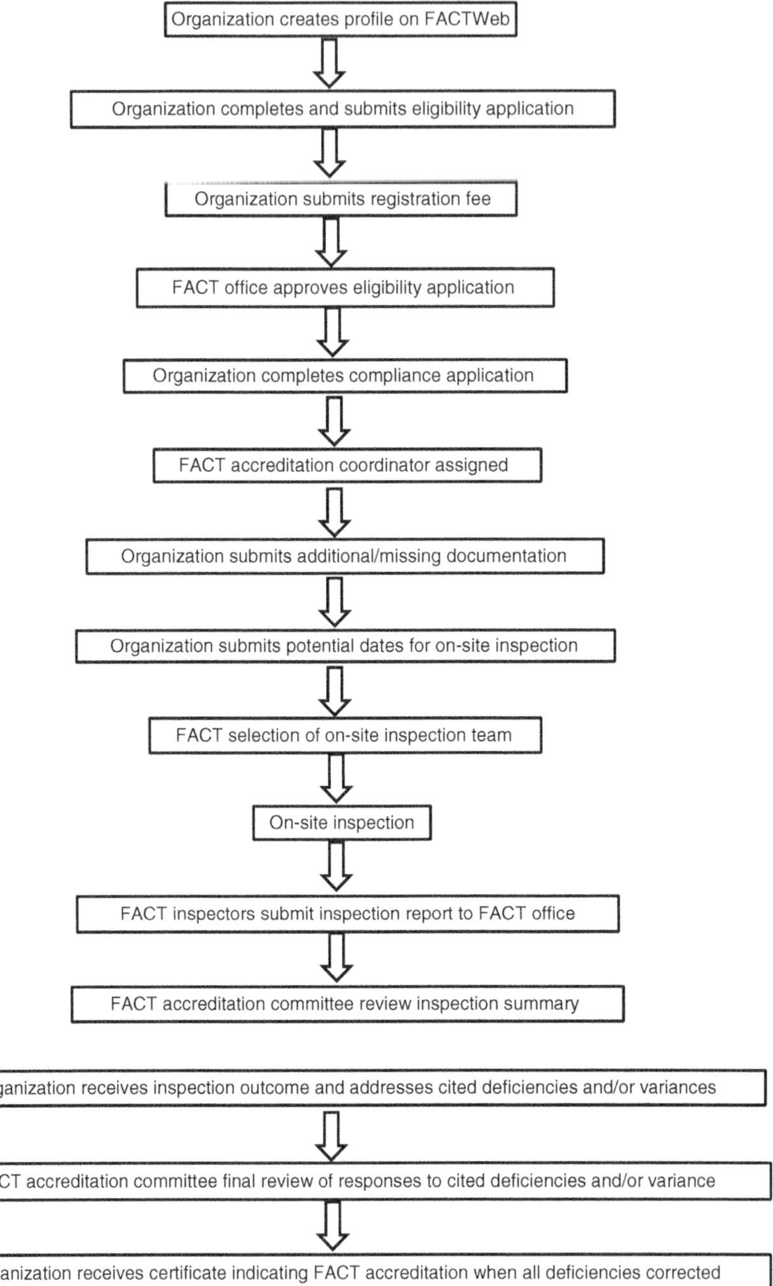

Fig. 2.1 FACT accreditation process

report to FACT after the on-site inspection. The FACT Accreditation Committee will review the inspection summary and submit a recommendation to the appropriate FACT Board. Significant questions, problems, and controversial or precedent-setting issues will be referred to the Board(s) for resolution. The organization director is then notified of the inspection outcome, and the organization is given a specified period of time to submit documentation addressing all cited deficiencies. The responses to the deficiencies are reviewed by the appropriate FACT Board that will then make a final determination. When all FACT Standards have been met, the organization receives a certificate indicating FACT accreditation (FACT n.d.). An annual report is required to be submitted to FACT for every year during the accreditation cycle. This annual report summarizes the activities of the program in the preceding year.

2.4.2 Joint Accreditation Committee-ISCT and EBMT

The Joint Accreditation Committee-ISCT and EBMT (JACIE) was cofounded in 1998 by both the European Group for Blood and Marrow Transplantation (EBMT) and ISCT (EBMT n.d.). It is a nonprofit accreditation organization that provides assessment and accreditation in the field of hematopoietic stem cell (HSC) transplantation. JACIE's primary aim is to promote high-quality patient care and laboratory performance in HSC collection, processing, and transplantation centers through the development of global standards and an internationally recognized system of accreditation (EBMT n.d.).

The initial accreditation process (Fig. 2.2) involves submitting a completed application form, signing the accreditation agreement with EBMT, and submitting a completed inspection checklist (JACIE n.d.-a). The form and checklist enable JACIE to determine if the organization is eligible for accreditation and to understand the structure of the organization and program as well as its relationship with other institutions.

Organizations seeking accreditation must submit pre-inspection documents before the actual inspection within 30 days from the receipt of the service agreement signed by the organization's representative to help the inspectors understand the organization's activities and to start checking compliance with some of the standards before the on-site visit. The requested documents include a selection of key SOPs, evidence of staff training and qualifications, official facility licenses and authorizations, quality management manual or handbook, basic evidence that the QM system is functioning, basic data on recent transplant activity, consent forms and related information, sample labels, plans or maps of the center, and sample agreements with third-party service providers (JACIE n.d.-b).

The on-site inspection usually lasts between 1 and 2 days (usually 1.5 days) depending on the size of the organization. During the inspection, the inspectors examine all aspects of the program in accordance with the accreditation checklist and verify the applicant's self-check. All staff members may be interviewed by the inspectors (JACIE n.d.-c). After the inspection, a final list of deficiencies is reported

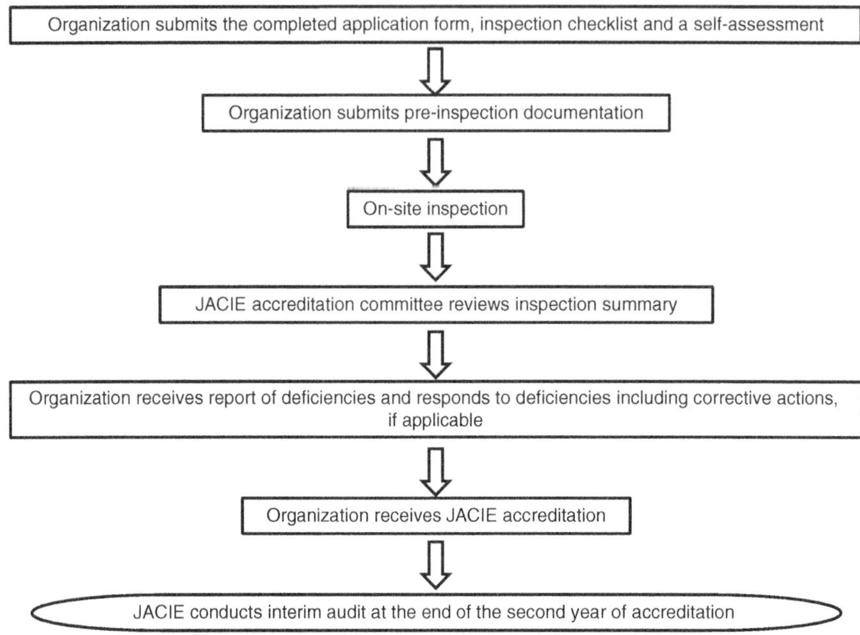

Fig. 2.2 JACIE accreditation process

to the organization, and responses including corrective action plans are expected. When all the responses are deemed appropriate, accreditation is conferred onto the organization.

Accredited organizations are required to submit an annual report to JACIE. The report should include a brief summary of important changes, if applicable, in the accredited organization and information relevant to transplantation and quality management (JACIE n.d.-d). An interim audit occurs at the end of the second year of accreditation. This audit focuses on the quality management system in the clinical units, collection, and processing facilities. The audit is conducted using the same edition of the Standards used for the preceding accreditation of the organization (JACIE n.d.-e).

2.4.3 American Association of Blood Banks (AABB)

AABB has developed standards for voluntary accreditation of hematopoietic progenitor cell (HPC), cord blood (CB), and other cellular therapy activities in addition to blood and blood components. AABB's accreditation program strives to improve the quality and safety of collecting, processing, testing, distributing, and administering cellular therapy products (AABB n.d.-a). AABB has been granted "deemed status" as an accrediting organization under the Clinical Laboratory Improvement Amendments of 1988 (CLIA 1988). Furthermore, the AABB accreditation program is accredited by the International Society for Quality in Healthcare (ISQua) (AABB n.d.-b).

AABB *Standards for Cellular Therapy Services* are revised every 2 years by the Cellular Therapy Standards Program Unit (CT SPU) that is comprised of individuals from the cellular therapy field including cord blood professionals, clinicians, medical and laboratory professionals, medical technologists, and quality experts (AABB 2013). The standards are organized into ten sections that focus on organization, resources, equipment, agreements, process control, documents and records, deviations and nonconforming products or services, internal and external assessments, process improvement, and safety and facilities. The facility's quality and operational systems are evaluated to ensure compliance with these standards as well as the CFR and CLIA 1988 (AABB n.d.-b).

For facilities to be accredited, they have to be in business for at least 6 months. The initial accreditation process is comprised of two phases, a self-assessment phase and an on-site assessment phase (Fig. 2.3). The self-assessment phase involves

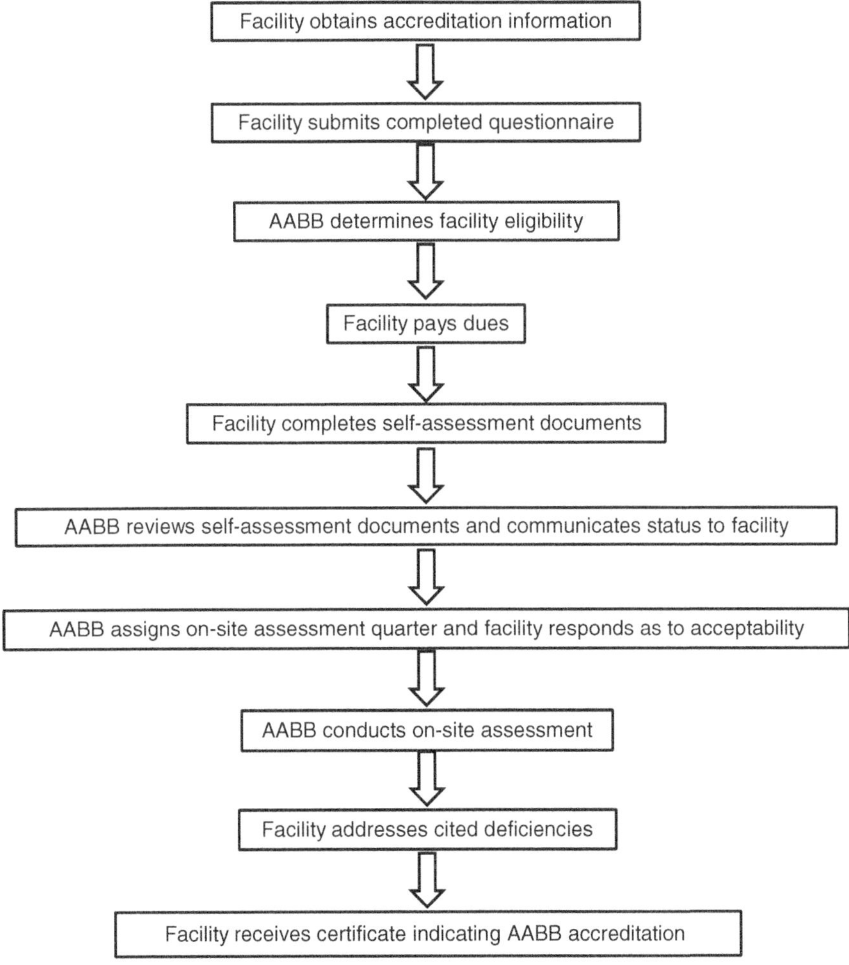

Fig. 2.3 AABB initial accreditation process

completing questionnaires/assessment tools for each activity; submitting policies, processes, procedures, labels, forms, lab workups, validation documents, and medical director information; and providing a quality plan overview. After the AABB National Office Accreditation Department reviews the documents, the facility is enrolled in the AABB Proficiency Testing Program and must pass at least five of six consecutive events prior to an on-site assessment. When the facility has satisfied all the requirements of the self-assessment phase, the AABB National Office Accreditation Department assigns a timeframe for the on-site assessment, the second phase (AABB n.d.-c). During the on-site assessment, trained AABB assessors who are highly skilled healthcare professionals from accredited organizations review the facility's operations for compliance with the latest edition of the AABB *Standards for Cellular Therapy Services*. Facilities are provided with the identity of the assessor in advance of the assessment for acceptance. Depending on the size and scope of activities performed by the facility, a team of assessors or one assessor may be assigned (AABB n.d.-b). Scheduled on-site assessments are conducted every 2 years. Upon completion of the assessment, the assessor/s will meet with staff to discuss the findings and leave a summary report of nonconformances with references to requirements. The facility is required to respond to all items listed as nonconformances by the due date on the summary report. The documents with the plan for corrective or preventive action will be reviewed by AABB and a decision made for granting accreditation (AABB n.d.-b).

AABB in conjunction with other nongovernmental organizations involved in cellular therapy developed the Circular of Information for the Use of Cellular Therapy Products. This document was also reviewed by the FDA and Health Resources and Service Administration. The Circular of Information is intended for users of certain minimally manipulated cellular therapy products including peripheral blood progenitor cells, bone marrow, cord blood, and leukocytes. A copy of this document can be found on AABB's website (AABB, America's Blood Centers et al. 2016).

2.4.4 College of American Pathologists (CAP)

The CAP Laboratory Accreditation Program (LAP) accredits all areas of the clinical laboratory in and out of the United States that perform testing on specimens from human beings or animals. CMS has granted the CAP LAP deeming authority, which allows a CAP inspection as a substitute for a CMS inspection. It is also recognized by The Joint Commission and can be used to meet many state certification requirements (CAP n.d.).

The CAP LAP uses a peer-based inspection model whereby teams of practicing professionals from a CAP-accredited institution are trained to conduct inspections. On-site inspections occur every 2 years using CAP accreditation checklists to assess compliance with program requirements (CAP n.d.). The checklists contain the accreditation program requirements which were developed through the expertise and collaboration between pathologists and laboratory professionals. The checklists are updated yearly to reflect current practices and technologies and are used by

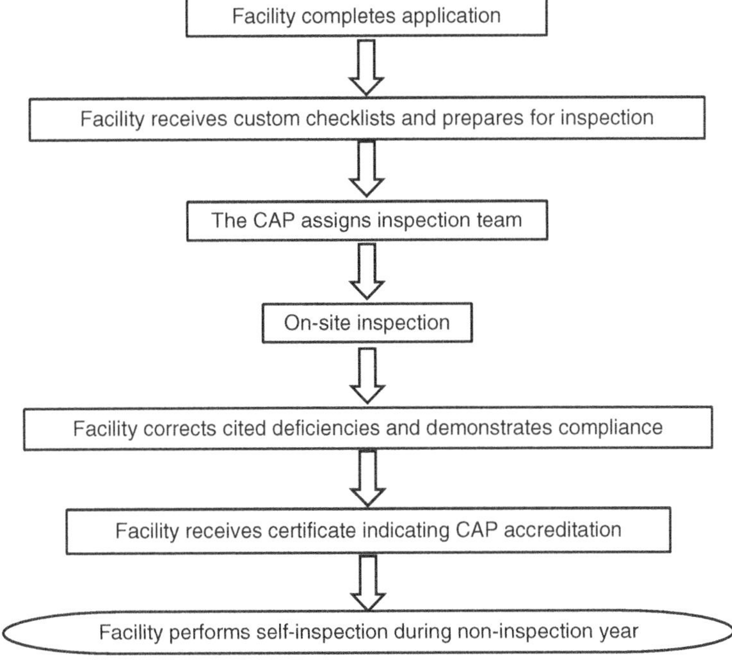

Fig. 2.4 CAP laboratory accreditation process

laboratories and inspectors to ensure quality and patient safety. Customized checklists based on the services offered by the laboratory/biorepository are provided for inspection preparation. The accreditation process is summarized in Fig. 2.4.

2.4.5 Other Accreditation Organizations

The World Marrow Donor Association (WMDA) is a voluntary organization that fosters international collaboration among blood stem cell donor registries, cord blood banks, and other organizations and individuals interested in blood stem cell transplantation (WMDA n.d.-a). Since January 1, 2017, the World Marrow Donor Association (WMDA), Bone Marrow Donors Worldwide (BMDW), and NetCord are one organization. WMDA provides a forum for discussion of various issues that relates to stem cell transplantation such as the clinical use of blood stem cells from unrelated donors across international boundaries and formulation of guidelines on logistics, quality control, ethics, finances, information technology, and registry accreditation (WMDA n.d.-a).

WMDA qualifies and accredits hematopoietic stem cell (HSC) donor registries that are used in the international search for an unrelated donor. Qualification and accreditation of these registries are an indication that these registries are committed to follow WMDA Standards. A two-step process was implemented in 2012 for accreditation. WMDA Qualified and WMDA Accredited are the first and second steps, respectively. After receiving accreditation, the organization is required to perform an internal self-evaluation every 2 years to become a WMNDA re-accredited organization (WMDA n.d.-b).

The National Marrow Donor Program (NMDP) is a nonprofit organization that operates the Be The Match Registry of volunteer hematopoietic stem cell donors and umbilical cord blood units in the United States. NMDP has established basic guidelines to facilitate hematopoietic cell transplants through its Standards. These requirements must be met by the partnering facility, its personnel, and its policies and procedures. The Standards have participation criteria for transplant centers, apheresis centers, collection centers, registries, and donor centers. The NMDP standards are designed to ensure that donors and patients receive high-quality care and that government standards are met. These Standards are reviewed every 2 years (NMDP n.d.).

The Health Resources and Services Administration (HRSA) within the Department of Health and Human Services oversees the C.W. Bill Young Cell Transplantation Program and the National Cord Blood Inventory for bone marrow and cord blood donations and transplant procedures coordinated by the National Marrow Donor Program.

The Alliance for Harmonization of Cellular Therapy Accreditation (AHCTA) is comprised of eight different organizations: (1) American Association of Blood Banks (AABB), (2) American Society for Blood and Marrow Transplantation (ASBMT), (3) European Group for Blood and Marrow Transplantation (EBMT), (4) Foundation for the Accreditation of Cellular Therapy (FACT), (5) International NetCord Foundation, (6) International Society for Cellular Therapy (Europe) (ISCT), (7) Joint Accreditation Committee-ISCT and EBMT (JACIE), and (8) World Marrow Donor Association (WMDA). The mission of this organization is to create a comprehensive single set of quality, safety, and professional requirements for cellular therapy that covers the process from assessment of donor eligibility to transplantation and clinical outcome. In order to achieve this goal, the member organizations have agreed to collaborate on the drafting of complementary standards and guidelines, to promote the concept of a global set of standards among the cellular therapy professional community and regulatory authorities, and to regularly communicate with each other on all relevant issues affecting cellular therapy guidelines. AHCTA partners with regulatory authorities in the application of these global standards which is important for their successful adoption and endeavors to inform and support these authorities in the area of cellular therapy regulation (ACHTA n.d.-a). The AHCTA website is a one-stop shop for resources such as the standards for the collaborating organizations (ACHTA n.d.-b). Crosswalk documents are also available that compare the different sets of cellular therapy standards for the collaborating organizations (ACHTA n.d.-a).

2.5 Expert Point of View

Cellular therapy processing laboratories are highly regulated by federal and state requirements to ensure the safety, purity, and potency of cellular therapy products. Processing laboratories should comply with FDA and CMS regulations as well as local state regulations at a minimum. While obtaining accreditation is not a federal requirement, it further improves the quality of a laboratory through compliance with its standards. Compliance with regulations and standards is verified through laboratory inspections. Having adequate facilities and equipment, highly trained and competent personnel, and a solid quality management plan is paramount to the successful operation of a processing laboratory. Regulations and standards are reviewed regularly by committees within each agency or organization, so it is important to keep abreast of changes. FDA, CMS, CDC, local state department of health, and accreditation organization websites provide useful resources for changes to regulations and standards and frequently asked questions.

2.6 Future Directions

As cellular therapies continue to be developed, the role of processing laboratories will expand from performing simple processing procedures to more complex manufacturing procedures. Regulations and standards governing the field of cellular therapy processing laboratories will continue to evolve as new innovations are developed for clinical use. As therapies previously in clinical trials become the standard of care, new regulations and standards need to be developed to ensure the continued safety, purity and potency of cellular therapies for patients. Processing laboratories will become more and more tightly regulated which will necessitate not only more resources from organizations to ensure a high quality of operations but also highly trained personnel. Transfusion medicine physicians with expertise in laboratory management will play an increasingly more important role in providing oversight of processing laboratories.

References

AABB, America's Blood Centers, the American Association of Tissue Banks, the American Red Cross, the American Society for Apheresis, the American Society for Blood and Marrow Transplantation, the College of American Pathologists, the Cord Blood Association, the Foundation for the Accreditation of Cellular Therapy, ICCBBA, the International Society for Cellular Therapy, the Joint Accreditation Committee of ISCT and EBMT, the National Marrow Donor Program, and Netcord (2016) Circular of information for the use of cellular therapy products. AABB, Bethesda, MD

AABB (n.d.-a) Accreditation program overview. http://www.aabb.org/sa/overview/Pages/default.aspx

AABB (n.d.-b) Accreditation program. http://www.aabb.org/sa/overview/Pages/program.aspx

AABB (n.d.-c) Become an AABB accredited facility (or add a new activity). http://www.aabb.org/sa/becomeaccredited/Pages/default.aspx

AABB AsBC, the American, Association of Tissue Banks tARC, the American Society for Apheresis, the, American Society for Blood and Marrow Transplantation tCoAP, the Cord Blood Association tFftAoCT, ICCBBA,, the International Society for Cellular Therapy tJACoI, and EBMT tNMDP, and Netcord (2016) Circular of information for the use of cellular therapy products. AABB, Bethesda, MD

ACHTA (n.d.-a) Documents. http://www.ahcta.org/docs/Mission%20statement%20AHTCA%20 FINAL.pdf

ACHTA (n.d.-b) Resources. http://www.ahcta.org/resources.html

CAP (n.d.) Laboratory accreditation program. http://www.cap.org/web/home/lab/accreditation /laboratory-accreditation-program?_afrLoop=402948075743307#!%40%40%3F_ afrLoop%3D402948075743307%26_adf.ctrl-state%3Dvy7a0e7fa_4

CDC (n.d.-a) Public health service act Sec 353. https://wwwn.cdc.gov/cliac/pdf/Addenda/ cliac0910/Addendum%20C_Yost.pdf

CDC (n.d.-b) Clinical laboratory improvement amendments (CLIA)—test complexities. https:// wwwn.cdc.gov/clia/resources/testcomplexities.aspx

CMS (n.d.-a) Clinical laboratory improvement amendments (CLIA). https://www.cms.gov/ Regulations-and-Guidance/Legislation/CLIA/index.html

CMS (n.d.-b) Proficiency testing programs. https://www.cms.gov/Regulations-and-Guidance/ Legislation/CLIA/Proficiency_Testing_Providers.html

CMS (n.d.-c) Clinical laboratory improvement amendments (CLIA). How to obtain a CLIA certificate. https://www.cms.gov/Regulations-and-Guidance/Legislation/CLIA/downloads/howobtaincliacertificate.pdf

CMS (n.d.-d) List of approved accreditation organizations under the clinical laboratory improvement amendments (CLIA). https://www.cms.gov/Regulations-and-Guidance/Legislation/ CLIA/Downloads/AOList.pdf

CMS (n.d.-e) Approved proficiency testing programs—2017. https://www.cms.gov/Regulations-and-Guidance/Legislation/CLIA/Downloads/ptlist.pdf

EBMT (n.d.) About JACIE. https://www.ebmt.org/Contents/Quality-Management/AboutJACIE/ Pages/About-JACIE.aspx

FACT (n.d.) Process overview. http://www.factwebsite.org/accreditationprocess/

FDA (n.d.) About FDA guidances. https://www.fda.gov/Drugs/%20GuidanceCompliance RegulatoryInformation/Guidances/default.htm

GPO (n.d.) Code of federal regulations. https://www.gpo.gov/fdsys/browse/collectionCfr. action?collectionCode=CFR

JACIE (n.d.-a) First-time application. http://www.jacie.org/applicants/first-time-application

JACIE(n.d.-b)Pre-inspectiondocumentshttp://www.jacie.org/applicants/pre-inspection-documents

JACIE (n.d.-c) The inspection. http://www.jacie.org/applicants/inspection

JACIE (n.d.-d) Annual report. http://www.jacie.org/applicants/annual-report

JACIE (n.d.-e) Interim audit. http://www.jacie.org/applicants/interim-audit

NMDP (n.d.) NMDP standards. https://bethematch.org/about-us/global-transplant-network/standards/

Rauch CA (2007) Laboratory accreditation and inspection. Clin Lab Med 27(4):845–858

The Joint Commission (n.d.) Facts about the Cooperative Accreditation Initiative https://www. jointcommission.org/facts_about_the_cooperative_accreditation_initiative/

U.S. Food and Drug Administration (n.d.-a) Tissue & tissue products. https://www.fda.gov/ BiologicsBloodVaccines/TissueTissueProducts/default.htm

U.S. Food and Drug Administration (n.d.-b) Minimal manipulation of human cells, tissues, and cellular and tissue-based products: draft guidance. https://www.fda.gov/BiologicsBloodVaccines/ GuidanceComplianceRegulatoryInformation/Guidances/CellularandGeneTherapy/ ucm427692.htm

U.S. Food and Drug Administration (n.d.-c) Registration and listing. https://www.fda.gov/forindustry/fdabasicsforindustry/ucm234625.htm

U.S. Food and Drug Administration (n.d.-d) What does FDA inspect? https://www.fda.gov/ AboutFDA/Transparency/basics/ucm194888.htm

U.S. Food and Drug Administration (n.d.-e) CLIA—clinical laboratory improvement amendments—currently waived analytes. https://www.accessdata.fda.gov/scripts/cdrh/cfdocs/ cfClia/analyteswaived.cfm

U.S. Food and Drug Administration (n.d.-f) CLIA—clinical laboratory improvement amendments search database https://www.accessdata.fda.gov/scripts/cdrh/cfdocs/cfCLIA/search.cfm

WMDA (n.d.-a) Who we are. https://www.wmda.info/about-us/who-we-are

WMDA (n.d.-b) WMDA accreditation programme

Part 1

HPC, Apheresis and HPC, Marrow

Donor Qualification for Hematopoietic Cell Transplantation

3

Patricia Shi

3.1 Introduction

Donor qualification assessment is a critical step in ensuring the safety and efficacy of the hematopoietic progenitor cell (HPC) transplantation process. Donor qualification refers to aspects of the donor that may affect safety of the donor, safety of the recipient, and success of the HPC transplantation in the recipient. This definition is synonymous with the term "donor suitability" used by the World Marrow Donor Association (WMDA) and American Association of Blood Banks (AABB). However, the term donor qualification is used for clarity because the term donor suitability can have different connotations in various contexts. For example, in FACT accreditation parlance, donor suitability is defined more narrowly as issues "that relate to the general health or medical fitness of the donor to undergo the collection procedure." In FDA parlance, in contrast, "donor suitability" is used interchangeably with "donor eligibility" or the infectious disease risk of the donor to recipient safety. The chapter provides an overview of the most important concepts in donor qualification assessment and a practical framework of how to systematically evaluate donor qualification.

3.2 Importance of Donor Qualification

Before a willing donor can proceed to donating a hematopoietic progenitor cell (HPC) product, the donor must be qualified. The purpose of donor qualification is to ensure safety of the donor and recipient, as well as safety and efficacy of the collected product. Although donor qualification is typically performed by the clinical

P. Shi
Lindsley F. Kimball Research Institute, New York Blood Center, New York, NY, USA
e-mail: PShi@nybc.org

J. Schwartz, B.H. Shaz (eds.), *Best Practices in Processing and Storage for Hematopoietic Cell Transplantation*, Advances and Controversies in Hematopoietic Transplantation and Cell Therapy,
https://doi.org/10.1007/978-3-319-58949-7_3

program, it is important for collection and processing facilities to understand the criteria used for proper donor qualification and document review of donor qualification. First, collection facilities must be informed of any medical issues in the donor impacting potential safety during the collection procedure. Second, collection facilities should confirm proper donor eligibility determination, and, in the event of an ineligible donor, collection and processing facilities must obtain urgent medical need documentation from the clinical program and ideally confirm both donor and recipient informed consent. Third, collection and processing facilities must label their products accordingly to eligibility determination data (or infectious disease testing for autologous donors). Lastly, for allogeneic donors, a summary of donor eligibility must accompany the HPC product whenever transported.

3.3 Basic Tenets of Donor Qualification

Donor qualification can be subdivided into three general considerations: (1) donor safety, (2) recipient safety, and (3) donor eligibility determination. The first, donor safety, applies to both autologous and allogeneic donors and assesses whether the donor can safely undergo the collection procedure. Thus, it focuses on the risk of the collection procedure to the donor's health. The latter two, recipient safety and donor eligibility, apply to allogeneic donors. Recipient safety assesses whether the donor has a medical condition—genetic, autoimmune, malignant, or infectious—which might be a risk to the intended recipient's health. Donor eligibility determination is a specific aspect of recipient safety, assessing the donor's potential to transmit an infectious disease to the recipient. This chapter is organized around these three issues. Human leukocyte antigen (HLA-A, HLA-B, HLA-C, and DRB1 is standard) matching between donor and recipient is critically important but is beyond the scope of this chapter; the reader is referred to guidelines published by organizations such as the National Marrow Donor Program or the Blood and Marrow Transplant Clinical Trials Network.

Donor qualification must be performed by healthcare providers with appropriate qualifications and training, and adequate knowledge of relevant federal regulations and accreditation requirements, to properly perform such assessments. Donor qualification must be performed prior to donor mobilization (as applicable) and recipient conditioning, but as close to the collection date as feasible, at maximum, within 90 days prior to collection. Donor blood testing for relevant communicable disease should be performed within 30 days prior to collection. The World Marrow Donor Association provides recommendations on maximum permissible intervals between assessment and collection (please see Table 3.5 at www.worldmarrow.org/donorsuitability).

3.4 Key Considerations During the Donor Qualification Process

A donor related to the recipient may be willing to accept a higher degree of personal risk related to donation than unrelated donors, which should be considered in evaluating donor risk: benefit ratio. Possible coercion, however, especially of related donors who may be under familial pressure to donate, must also be prevented by having a qualified health provider other than the recipient's transplant physician obtain informed consent.

Although a donor typically undergoes full informed consent later in the qualification process, it is important to perform donor education and medical screening at the time of recruitment or immediately prior to HLA typing in order to gauge donor willingness and appropriateness, clearly delineate expectations, and expeditiously defer any ineligible donors. Donors must be made aware that they are expected to share information about personal health issues that potentially affect recipient safety. By discussing donor and recipient safety issues up front, potential delays to transplant or potential guilt of donors who are HLA-matched but not otherwise eligible due to lifestyle or medical conditions can be avoided. The World Marrow Donor Association has recommendations on the minimum donor information that should be requested at sequential stages of qualification (refer to Tables 3.1, 3.2 and 3.3 at www.worldmarrow.org/donorsuitability).

There are many required elements to proper informed consent, a discussion of which are beyond the scope of this chapter. The reader is referred to FDA regulations (CFR 21, Chapter I, Part 50) as well as accreditation organization standards (FACT/JACIE (Joint Accreditation Committee-ISCT & EBMT), AABB) for further details (see Chap. 2). At minimum, informed consent should describe the risks and benefits of the collection process and procedure, its relevance and consequences of refusal to the potential recipient, short- and long-term risks and side effects of donation, required testing, donor rights and confidentiality, communication and sharing of donor qualification data, insurance coverage for possible adverse events, the possibility of future donation requests, and rights to and ownership of the collected product.

3.5 Evaluation of Donor Safety

Donor safety assesses whether the donor can safely undergo the collection procedure. Donor safety criteria, especially for unrelated donors, are generally stringent because HPC donation is an altruistic act. A licensed healthcare professional should perform a comprehensive assessment of donor safety within 90 days prior to collection that includes review of current and past health issues, medications and allergies, physical exam, and lab testing. Certain donor safety evaluations are required by accreditation organizations (Table 3.1). Importantly, for allogeneic donors, the healthcare provider evaluating donor safety cannot be the same one primarily responsible for care of the recipient, due to conflict of interest. Furthermore for allo geneic donors, an independent donor advocate should be available, especially for minors or people with mental disabilities (Bitan et al. 2016; van Walraven et al. 2010). Although standard for unrelated donors, ensuring impartiality of the donor safety evaluation is especially relevant for related donors since, in light of the efficacy, safety, and availability of fully HLA-matched sibling donor (MSD) transplant, donor safety criteria tend to be more flexible than for unrelated donors (Worel et al. 2015).

Table 3.1 Donor safety requirements for hematopoietic progenitor cell donors

Accreditation organization	Donor safety requirements for HPC donors
FACT/JACIE and AABB	–Defined donor qualification criteria, including for pediatric and elderly donors –Donor safety determination: for allogeneic donors, by a licensed health care professional not directly involved in recipient care –Written assessment of donor safety performed by a qualified health care professional immediately prior to each collection procedure –Complete blood count with platelet count within 24 h prior to each subsequent collection procedure
FACT/JACIE	–Donor advocate for allogeneic donors who are minors or mentally incapacitated –Defined minimal peripheral blood count criteria to proceed with the collection procedure
AABB	–Access to donor advocate for all allogeneic donors –Defined criteria for discontinuation of collection due to medical complications

FACT Foundation for the Accreditation of Cellular Therapy, *JACIE* Joint Accreditation Committee-ISCT and EBMT, *AABB* American Association of Blood Banks

Importantly, focused evaluation of donor safety should periodically continue after initial donor qualification, as donor circumstances may change. Indeed, FACT/JACIE and AABB require an update of donor safety issues by a qualified healthcare professional immediately prior to each collection (see Chaps. 1 and 2). In order to assist with qualification of donors with medical health issues, the World Marrow Donor Association established and maintains recommended acceptance criteria for many medical conditions at www.worldmarrow.org/donorsuitability (World Marrow Donor Association Clinical Working Group C 2016). If a donor does have significant medical issues, a specialist familiar with the process and risks of the donation procedure should be consulted to determine if a more than minimally increased risk over the baseline safety profile of the HPC collection procedure exists.

HPC collection can be accomplished by either bone marrow (BM) harvest or peripheral blood (PB) $CD34^+$ cell (hematopoietic progenitor cell-apheresis [HPC-apheresis]) collection, and certain aspects of donor safety are specific to each collection procedure type (Table 3.2). For BM collection, there are risks from the surgical procedure and its associations such as anesthesia, and with HPC-Apheresis collection, there are risks from the apheresis procedure(s) and mobilization agents such as G-CSF. Although serious adverse events (SAEs) are less frequent and donor recovery is shorter with HPC, Apheresis compared to BM collection, <1% of donors of either type of collection (BM or PB) experience SAE (Burns et al. 2016; Pulsipher et al. 2014; Halter et al. 2009). There are higher incidences of donation-associated adverse events with obesity (BMI > 40), older age, and female gender (Pulsipher et al. 2013). In general, allogeneic donors must have stable and good mental and physical health, especially unrelated donors. Female donors cannot be pregnant,

Table 3.2 Recommended donor safety determination by type of collection procedure

Procedure type	History and physical	Other assessment
BM and PB hematopoietic progenitor cell collection	Pregnancy; acute medical conditions; significant cardiac, cerebrovascular, renal, or pulmonary disease	CBC with differential, Chem 20, pregnancy screen (within 7 days of collection), urinalysis, type and screen Optional: CXR, EKG
BM collection only	Serious neck, back, spine, or hip conditions/surgery; oropharyngeal disease; obstructive sleep apnea; potential need for red cell transfusion; bleeding risk/condition	American Society of Anesthesiologists Physical Status (ASA-PS) classification system
PB progenitor cell collection only	Need for and risk with central venous access placement, sickle cell disease or other hemoglobinopathies, splenomegaly, breastfeeding, autoimmune disease, inflammatory eye conditions, deep venous thrombosis or pulmonary embolism risk, thrombocytopenia <150,000/μl, significant liver disease, lithium use	Optional but suggested: hemoglobin fractionation

and breastfeeding should be halted during anesthetic, G-CSF, or plerixafor administration. FACT/JACIE Standards require that pregnancy testing be performed within 7 days prior to starting the donor mobilization regimen and also within 7 days prior to initiation of the recipient's preparative regimen.

BM harvest is the operative extraction of bone marrow, typically under general anesthesia, through multiple punctures of the cortical bone, most commonly the iliac crest. An individual's preoperative physical status can be assessed using the American Society of Anesthesiologists Physical Status (ASA-PS) classification system (Hackett et al. 2015; American Society of Anesthesiologists 2014). People with pre-existing cardiac ischemia, heart failure, cerebrovascular disease, insulin-dependent diabetes mellitus, or renal dysfunction are at higher risk of adverse events with general anesthesia (Kristensen et al. 2014; Fleisher et al. 2014). People with pre-existing neurologic, cardiovascular, or pulmonary issues are also at risk for long-term cognitive dysfunction with general anesthesia, so their safety deserves careful consideration by a disease specialist familiar with the collection procedure. Donors with serious oropharyngeal, neck, back, spine, or hip conditions; abnormal platelet function; or malignant hyperthermia should be precluded due to the risks of anesthesia; potential bone, nerve, or vessel damage; and bleeding. A high recipient to donor blood volume may require a relatively high volume of bone marrow to be collected; in such cases, preoperative autologous donation should be considered to avoid potential allogeneic red cell transfusion.

HPC, Apheresis collection is the collection of HPC through apheresis after mobilizing HPC from the BM into the PB via the subcutaneous administration most commonly of G-CSF for 4–5 days and sometimes with plerixafor (in autologous setting only). A normal baseline platelet count is desirable because large volume leukapheresis can significantly lower the platelet count. The risk of potential central venous catheter placement must be evaluated, especially in younger donors who may require general anesthesia. Plerixafor is primarily cleared by the kidneys and should be dose-reduced by one third in patients with creatinine clearance ≤50 ml/min. Administration of G-CSF also requires specific considerations. Potential donors must be screened for sickle cell disease because G-CSF can cause life-threatening vaso-occlusion. Not all patients with sickle cell disease are symptomatic, so although hemoglobin fractionation is not required, it is suggested. Although the G-CSF package insert also asserts contraindication in sickle cell trait, literature suggests G-CSF mobilization is safe with trait (Kang et al. 2002; Panch et al. 2016). G-CSF can cause splenic enlargement and rarely rupture, so donors with preexisting splenomegaly, such as with thalassemia, need to be carefully evaluated. G-CSF can precipitate inflammatory eye disease (Parkkali et al. 1996; Tsuchiyama et al. 2000) and gout (Spitzer et al. 1998), exacerbate autoimmune disorders (Snowden et al. 2012; Kroschinsky et al. 2004), and elevate serum alkaline phosphatase and LDH. Drug interactions between lithium and G-CSF may exacerbate the neutrophilia observed with G-CSF alone. G-CSF may cause transient hypercoagulability, so donors with a history or risk of venous thrombosis or pulmonary embolism may need venous thromboembolism prophylaxis. G-CSF can cause hematuria and glomerulonephritis (Pulsipher et al. 2014; Lee et al. 2016), so donors with hematuria on urinalysis or known immune nephropathy may require exclusion. G-CSF can cause acute respiratory distress syndrome and alveolar hemorrhage, so donors with significant respiratory conditions should probably be excluded. Evidence suggests that there is no increased risk of malignancy with G-CSF administration; long-term follow-up of pediatric donors receiving G-CSF is currently being studied, but no data to date suggest concern.

3.6 Evaluation of Recipient Safety

Recipient safety applies to allogeneic donors and assesses whether the donor has a medical condition, such as infectious, genetic, autoimmune, or malignant disease, which might be a risk to the intended recipient's health. Qualification of donors in regard to recipient safety is less stringent than qualification in regard to donor safety, due to the often life-threatening nature of the recipient's condition. Furthermore, the recipient's primary transplant provider, in contrast to donor safety considerations, is critically involved in recipient safety considerations.

Careful personal and family medical histories, physical exam, and routine lab tests are required to determine recipient safety (Table 3.3). Chest x-ray, electrocardiogram, and other tests like echocardiograms or abdominal ultrasounds may be indicated if there is a specific rationale for testing. Donors <60 years of age are preferable due to increased frequency with age of chronic, serious disease and the higher quality of HPCs from younger donors. Donors with psychiatric disorders must be assessed for their capacity to adhere to the donation process. Donors with any history of radiation or chemotherapy may transmit risk of future myelodysplasia. Recipient development of the same autoimmune disease of a donor is well reported. Thus, most centers would exclude donors with a history of hematologic or invasive solid malignancy, symptomatic congenital blood disease or immunodeficiency (versus a carrier state), Down syndrome, or systemic multi-organ autoimmune disorder. In regard to infectious disease, donors with HIV or any type of Creutzfeldt-Jakob disease (CJD) are typically excluded. All HPC donor-derived malignancies so far reported have been hematologic (Lown et al. 2014). Thus, related donors, especially with abnormal blood counts, should be carefully evaluated to rule out inherited predisposition to hematopoietic malignancy or potential for malignancy (Churpek et al. 2012; Xiao et al. 2011; Babushok et al. 2016).

In order to assist with qualification of donors with medical health issues, the World Marrow Donor Association established and maintains recommended acceptance criteria for many medical conditions affecting recipient safety at www.worldmarrow.org/donorsuitability (World Marrow Donor Association Clinical Working Group C 2016).

Although perhaps not typically regarded as a recipient safety issue, it is also important to perform ABO/Rh and red blood cell antibody screening on allogeneic donors, in order to determine and mitigate risk to the recipient of major and minor ABO incompatibility and alloimmune red cell hemolysis complications.

Table 3.3 Allogeneic donor screening for recipient safety

Procedure type	History and physical	Blood test
BM and PB hematopoietic progenitor cell collection	–Inherited disease –Malignant, hematologic, immunologic , or autoimmune disease –Radiation or chemotherapy –Psychiatric disorder –Drug or alcohol addiction –Donor eligibility determination (travel, high-risk behavior, blood transfusion, organ or xenotransplant, vaccinations, medications)	–CBC with diff, Chem 20, urinalysis, type and screen –Optional: SPEP, coagulation screen, ESR, blood smear review –Infectious disease testing (within 30 days before HPC or 7 days of MNC/donor lymphocyte)

CBC complete blood count, *SPEP* serum protein electrophoresis, *ESR* sedimentation rate, *HPC* hematopoietic progenitor cell, *MNC* mononuclear cell

3.7 Determining Donor Eligibility

Donor eligibility determination is a specific aspect of recipient safety, assessing the donor's potential to transmit a relevant infectious disease to the recipient. Determination is required by the FDA since May 2005, with the most current regulations specified in the Code of Federal Regulations (CFR) in Title 21, Part 1271, Subpart C (http://www.ecfr.gov). Detailed guidance on how to comply with donor eligibility requirements was released in August 2007 "Eligibility Determination for Donors of Human Cells, Tissues, and Cellular and Tissue-Based Products (HCT/Ps)." This guidance was recently supplemented with "Revised Recommendations for Determining Eligibility of Donors of Human Cells, Tissues, and Cellular and Tissue-Based Products Who Have Received Human-Derived Clotting Factor Concentrates" published November 2016 (www.fda.gov/BiologicsBloodVaccines/GuidanceComplianceRegulatoryInformation/Guidances/Tissue/).

Donor qualification in respect to eligibility determination has some flexibility; even if a donor is ineligible or the determination incomplete, the donor can still donate and the product distributed with documentation of urgent medical need by the clinical program. Urgent medical need is defined as a situation in which no comparable cellular therapy product is available and the recipient is likely to suffer death or serious morbidity without the cellular therapy product.

Donor eligibility determination is based on results of donor screening and donor testing. Screening determines that the donor has no risk factors or clinical evidence of infection with "relevant" communicable disease agents, with relevance typically being established by national competent authorities such as the FDA. Communicable disease agents currently considered relevant in the USA are listed in Table 3.4. Relevant communicable disease agents may have region-specific requirements based on disease endemicity. Donor testing is laboratory testing of donor blood for evidence of relevant infectious disease agents. In the USA, blood tests specifically licensed, cleared, or approved by the FDA must be used, and testing must be performed by a laboratory certified under the Clinical Laboratory Improvement Amendments (CLIA) of 1988 or meeting equivalent requirements as determined by the Centers for Medicare and Medicaid Services (also see Chap. 2).

For screening, the FDA requires review of "relevant medical records." Relevant medical records are defined as the following: (1) history questionnaire (current medical history and relevant social behavior interview), (2) current relevant physical exam, (3) laboratory test results (other than for eligibility determination), (4) available medical records, and (5) any other information pertaining to risk factors for relevant communicable disease, such as social behavior, clinical signs and symptoms of relevant communicable disease, and treatments related to medical conditions suggestive of risk for relevant communicable disease. For subsequent donations within 6 months of the comprehensive donor screening, an abbreviated screening focused on changes in donor medical history and relevant social history may be performed.

Identification of donor risk factors is critical. For example, travel history to areas endemic for malaria, West Nile virus, Zika, Chagas, and variant Creutzfeldt-Jakob disease must be identified. As another example, sexual intimacy with: people

Table 3.4 Relevant communicable diseases

Evaluation required by FDA regulation	HIV-1 and HIV-2	HQ[a], PE[a], blood test
	HTLV-I and HTLV-II	HQ, PE, blood test
	Hepatitis B	HQ, PE, blood test
	Hepatitis C	HQ, PE, blood test
	CMV[b]	blood test
	Human transmissible spongiform encephalopathy (e.g., any type of Creutzfeldt-Jakob disease)	HQ
	Treponema pallidum (syphilis)	HQ, blood test
Evaluation required by FDA guidance	West Nile virus	HQ, PE, blood test
	Zika virus	HQ, PE
	Sepsis (includes bacteremia)	HQ, PE
	Vaccinia virus (smallpox)	HQ, PE
Not FDA required but instituted by others (e.g., NMDP, FACT/JACIE)	*Trypanosoma cruzi* (Chagas disease)	HQ, blood test
	Malaria, tuberculosis	HQ
	Epstein-Barr virus, *Toxoplasma gondii*, varicella zoster virus, Herpes simplex virus	Blood tests

[a]*HQ* history questionnaire, *PE* physical exam
[b]Required by the FDA but not regarded as a relevant communicable disease; donor eligibility is determined by the transplanting facility

with hepatitis, male travelers to areas with active Zika virus transmission, or xenotransplantation recipients must be identified. FDA requirements regarding risk factors or conditions to be screened for are specific and detailed; thus, the use of a donor history questionnaire developed by a professional organization is strongly recommended. It is important to note that there are some differences between FDA requirements for blood donors and HPC donors. With this in mind, an interorganizational task force has developed a HPC-specific health history questionnaire that is regularly updated to reflect the latest FDA and accreditation requirements; it can be found at www.aabb.org/tm/questionnaires/Pages/dhqhpc.aspx or http://www.factwebsite.org/Inner.aspx?id=163.

Likewise, screening also includes physical exam, as certain symptoms and signs of infectious disease risk- for example, needle marks, tattoos, weight loss, night sweats, fever, cough, shortness of breath, jaundice, hepatomegaly, lymphadenopathy, mouth or skin lesions, and rash- may only be detected by clinical exam. Section IV, parts F and G of the FDA's August 2007 Donor Eligibility Guidance provides detailed information as to specific physical exam evidence that should be screened for to meet 21 CFR 1271.75 regulations.

Finally, donor eligibility determination requires laboratory testing of donor blood for relevant infectious diseases, since donors with relevant communicable disease can often by asymptomatic. Such testing is typically governed by national competent authorities. The WMDA has released recommendations on minimum standards for infectious disease testing (Table 3.4 at www.worldmarrow.org/donorsuitability). The FDA allows specimens for communicable disease testing to be collected up to 30 days prior to or 7 days after HPC collection; if collected after HPC collection, issues of test accuracy related to plasma dilution due to transfusion or intravenous fluid infusion apply (Part 1271, Subpart C, 1271.80); it is thus recommended to avoid these complexities by drawing the sample prior to the collection procedure. The FDA lists current FDA-licensed donor screening tests at www.fda.gov/cber/products/testkits.htm.

An eligibility determination statement and a summary of the records used to make the determination must be provided by all distributors of allogeneic HCT/P products. If donor eligibility is incomplete or the donor is ineligible, the reason/s must be documented and incomplete or positive screening or testing clearly specified. The HCT/P product cannot be transferred or released without documentation of urgent medical need.

3.8 Other Aspects of Donor Qualification

It is worthwhile to note that national competent authorities may have country-specific regulations of, and parlance for, HPC products (Table 3.5). For example, currently, specific HPC product types are differentially regulated by the FDA (Table 3.6). The FDA regulates "minimally manipulated" peripheral blood HPCs that are autologous or family related (first or second degree relative) as "361 products" that are regulated under 21 CFR 1271 and Section 361 of the Public Health Services Act, whereas unrelated HPCs, whether minimally manipulated or not and even autologous or family-related HPCs that are more than minimally manipulated, are regulated as drug or biologic products under Section 351 of the PHS Act. All HPC collection facilities (unless solely under contract by an FDA-registered facility) and processing facilities must register with FDA, annually update their registration, and annually submit to FDA a list of each HCT/P manufactured.

Table 3.5 Glossary of key FDA definitions

Term	Definition
Human cells, tissues, and cellular and tissue-based products (HCT/P)	Articles containing or consisting of human cells or tissues that are intended for implantation, transplantation, infusion, or transfer into a human recipient. All peripheral blood HPC products, but not minimally manipulated bone marrow products, are considered HCT/P.
Manufacture	Any or all steps in the recovery, processing, storage, labeling, packaging, or distribution of any human cell or tissue, and the screening or testing of the cell or tissue donor.
Recovery	Collection of HCT/P.

Table 3.6 Regulations for minimally manipulated human cell tissue product

Donor	Marrow	Peripheral blood
Autologous	No federal regulation	Section 361 of the PHS Act 21 CFR 1271, except Subpart C, donor eligibility (recommended but not required)
Related allogeneic	No federal regulation	Section 361 of the PHS Act 21 CFR 1271
Unrelated allogeneic	Division of Transplantation within the Health Resources and Service Administration	Regulated as drug, device, and/or biological product under Section 351 of the PHS Act 21 CFR Subchapters C and H 21 CFR 1271 Subparts C and D

3.9 Expert Point of View

Proper and complete donor qualification assessment is constantly changing, due to continually emerging new transmissible disease risks and continual new data on noninfectious donor conditions that may affect donor safety or recipient safety. Interested parties are encouraged to keep updated on latest developments as provided by the WMDA, accreditation bodies such as FACT/JACIE and AABB, and their national competent authorities. For example, the FDA has a free e-mail alert service for receipt of important FDA news and documents, such as guidances, as they become available (sign up at www.fda.gov/AboutFDA/ContactFDA/StayInformed/GetEmailUpdates). The WMDA welcomes requests for review of individual medical conditions from all those with responsibility for HPC donors, related or unrelated (contact info can be found at www.worldmarrow.org/donorsuitability). FACT/JACIE and AABB also encourage feedback or clarification on existing accreditation standards as well as suggestions for new standards. The Cellular Therapy Committee at AABB also has a subcommittee specifically devoted to (US) regulatory affairs which can be joined at www.aabb.org/membership/governance/committees/Pages/ctsubsections.aspx#ra.

3.10 Future Directions

This chapter has introduced multiple resources available to assist with donor suitability assessment. Donor eligibility assessment by medical history and relevant social behavior interview has been significantly simplified by the development and maintenance of an HPC-specific health history questionnaire and associated materials (www.aabb.org/tm/questionnaires/Pages/dhqhpc.aspx) by a task force comprised of representatives from AABB, the American Association of Tissue Banks, the American Society for Blood and Marrow Transplantation, the American Society for Apheresis, FACT, JACIE, the International Society for Cellular Therapy, and NMDP; an FDA liaison; and an ethicist.

Future directions might be for consensus task forces to develop similar specific questionnaire materials for donor safety and recipient safety assessment that are also regularly updated with the latest safety data. Although guidance is available, particularly from the WMDA, specific questionnaire-driven algorithms have yet to be developed. Donor safety questionnaire/s should incorporate apheresis-specific versus BM-specific issues. The recipient safety questionnaire should cover donor genetic, autoimmune, and malignant conditions, as well as relevant infectious disease conditions outside of donor eligibility requirements.

Furthermore, databases could be developed to correlate donor medical conditions affecting donor and recipient safety with donor and recipient adverse events and long-term outcomes. Although such databases are already developed by organizations involved in unrelated donor recruitment such as the NMDP, these donors are typically healthy. A similar adverse event identification and long-term follow-up of related donors on an epidemiologic rather than case report level is needed. A consensus statement on a minimum data set for prospective donor follow-up has been published by the Worldwide Network for Blood and Marrow Transplantation (Halter et al. 2013).

References

American Society of Anesthesiologists (2014) ASA physical status classification system

Babushok DV, Bessler M, Olson TS (2016) Genetic predisposition to myelodysplastic syndrome and acute myeloid leukemia in children and young adults. Leuk Lymphoma 57(3):520–536

Bitan M et al (2016) Determination of eligibility in related pediatric hematopoietic cell donors: ethical and clinical considerations. Recommendations from a Working Group of the Worldwide Network for Blood and Marrow Transplantation Association. Biol Blood Marrow Transplant 22(1):96–103

Burns LJ et al (2016) Recovery of unrelated donors of peripheral blood stem cells versus recovery of unrelated donors of bone marrow: a prespecified analysis from the phase III blood and marrow transplant clinical trials network protocol 0201. Biol Blood Marrow Transplant 22(6):1108–1116

Churpek JE et al (2012) Identifying familial myelodysplastic/acute leukemia predisposition syndromes through hematopoietic stem cell transplantation donors with thrombocytopenia. Blood 120(26):5247–5249

Fleisher LA et al (2014) 2014 ACC/AHA guideline on perioperative cardiovascular evaluation and management of patients undergoing noncardiac surgery: a report of the American College of Cardiology/American Heart Association task force on practice guidelines. J Am Coll Cardiol 64(22):e77–137

Hackett NJ, De Oliveira GS, Jain UK, Kim JY (2015) ASA class is a reliable independent predictor of medical complications and mortality following surgery. Int J Surg 18:184–190

Halter J et al (2009) Severe events in donors after allogeneic hematopoietic stem cell donation. Haematologica 94(1):94–101

Halter JP et al (2013) Allogeneic hematopoietic stem cell donation-standardized assessment of donor outcome data: a consensus statement from the Worldwide Network for Blood and Marrow Transplantation (WBMT). Bone Marrow Transplant 48(2):220–225

Kang EM et al (2002) Mobilization, collection, and processing of peripheral blood stem cells in individuals with sickle cell trait. Blood 99(3):850–855

Kristensen SD et al (2014) 2014 ESC/ESA guidelines on non-cardiac surgery: cardiovascular assessment and management: the joint task force on non-cardiac surgery: cardiovascular assessment and management of the European Society of Cardiology (ESC) and the European Society of Anaesthesiology (ESA). Eur Heart J 35(35):2383–2431

Kroschinsky F et al (2004) Severe autoimmune hyperthyroidism after donation of growth factor-primed allogeneic peripheral blood progenitor cells. Haematologica 89(4):ECR05

Lee JB et al (2016) Exacerbation of IgA nephropathy following G-CSF administration for PBSC collection: suggestions for better donor screening. Bone Marrow Transplant 51(2):286–287

Lown RN et al (2014) Unrelated adult stem cell donor medical suitability: recommendations from the World Marrow Donor Association Clinical Working Group Committee. Bone Marrow Transplant 49(7):880–886

Panch SR et al (2016) Hematopoietic progenitor cell mobilization is more robust in healthy African American compared to Caucasian donors and is not affected by the presence of sickle cell trait. Transfusion 56(5):1058–1065

Parkkali T, Volin L, Siren MK, Ruutu T (1996) Acute iritis induced by granulocyte colony-stimulating factor used for mobilization in a volunteer unrelated peripheral blood progenitor cell donor. Bone Marrow Transplant 17(3):433–434

Pulsipher MA et al (2013) Acute toxicities of unrelated bone marrow versus peripheral blood stem cell donation: results of a prospective trial from the National Marrow Donor Program. Blood 121(1):197–206

Pulsipher MA et al (2014) Lower risk for serious adverse events and no increased risk for cancer after PBSC vs BM donation. Blood 123(23):3655–3663

Snowden JA et al (2012) Haematopoietic SCT in severe autoimmune diseases: updated guidelines of the European Group for Blood and Marrow Transplantation. Bone Marrow Transplant 47(6):770–790

Spitzer T, McAfee S, Poliquin C, Colby C (1998) Acute gouty arthritis following recombinant human granulocyte colony-stimulating factor therapy in an allogeneic blood stem cell donor. Bone Marrow Transplant 21(9):966–967

Tsuchiyama J et al (2000) Recurrent idiopathic iridocyclitis after autologous peripheral blood stem-cell transplantation followed by G-CSF administration for acute lymphoblastic leukemia. Ann Hematol 79(5):269–271

van Walraven SM et al (2010) Family donor care management: principles and recommendations. Bone Marrow Transplant 45(8):1269–1273

Worel N et al (2015) Suitability criteria for adult related donors: a consensus statement from the worldwide network for blood and marrow transplantation standing committee on donor issues. Biol Blood Marrow Transplant 21(12):2052–2060

World Marrow Donor Association Clinical Working Group C (2016) WMDA donor medical suitability recommendations

Xiao H et al (2011) First report of multiple CEBPA mutations contributing to donor origin of leukemia relapse after allogeneic hematopoietic stem cell transplantation. Blood 117(19):5257–5260

Routine Hematopoietic Progenitor Cell Processing: HPC, Apheresis and HPC, Marrow Products

4

Jay S. Raval, Kathryn McKay, and Yara A. Park

4.1 Introduction: Why This Chapter Is Important

Upon collection of hematopoietic progenitor cells (HPCs), there are numerous steps that must take place to guarantee the potency and purity of the product in anticipation of transplantation. Every HPC product must have cell enumeration, flow cytometric immunophenotypic studies, sterility testing, viability studies, and, if necessary, cryopreservation and storage. It is critical that cryopreserved HPC products that may be stored for up to years be done so in a way that permits the cells to remain viable and functional in order for engraftment to occur after transplantation. In this chapter, laboratory processes specifically pertaining to HPC, Apheresis and HPC, Marrow products will be discussed. In addition, we will discuss the indications and associated matters for HPC product manipulation of both autologous and allogeneic products that are collected by either apheresis technology or bone marrow harvest. More detailed information about HPC laboratory regulation and accreditation is reviewed in Chap. 2.

4.2 Following the Rules: Regulation and Accreditation

HPC products are considered biologics; thus, the laboratories that process these unique products are highly regulated and must be registered or licensed with the US Food and Drug Administration (FDA) for the use of these products in the USA. If

J.S. Raval, M.D. (✉) • Y.A. Park, M.D.
Department of Pathology and Laboratory Medicine, University of North Carolina at Chapel Hill, Chapel Hill, NC, USA
e-mail: jay_raval@med.unc.edu

K. McKay, M.S., M.T. (A.S.C.P.)
Advanced Cellular Therapeutics Facility, UNC Lineberger Comprehensive Cancer Center, Chapel Hill, NC, USA

J. Schwartz, B.H. Shaz (eds.), *Best Practices in Processing and Storage for Hematopoietic Cell Transplantation*, Advances and Controversies in Hematopoietic Transplantation and Cell Therapy,
https://doi.org/10.1007/978-3-319-58949-7_4

these facilities are Clinical Laboratory Improvement Amendments (CLIA) certified, then FDA regulations, state laws, and/or College of American Pathologists (CAP) guidelines are followed. Additionally, laboratory accreditation by the AABB (formerly known as the American Association of Blood Banks) and the Foundation for the Accreditation of Cellular Therapy (FACT) is often obtained.

Regardless of whether the product is apheresis or marrow derived, these products often require at least minimal analysis and manipulation to guarantee safety and efficacy.

4.3 Autologous HPC Products: The Donor Is the Recipient

The overwhelming majority of autologous HPC products are collected by apheresis technology. Autologous HPC products do not have issues involving ABO incompatibilities, as the donor and recipient are the same. However, a collected autologous HPC product may not be infused immediately and could require preservation until the patient has been prepared and deemed ready for hematopoietic cell transplantation. Each HPC product is aliquoted into storage bags based on predetermined total nucleated cell (TNC) concentrations, after which point a cryoprotectant is added prior to the freezing process. Samples for sterility testing are usually collected immediately subsequent to the addition of cryoprotectant but antecedent to cryopreservation.

4.3.1 Optimizing Cell Concentrations: How Much Is Enough?

The optimal TNC concentration for use during HPC product cryopreservation is currently unknown. Poor mobilizers are typically defined as (a) not having achieved a circulating $CD34^+$ count >20/μl within 6 days after G-CSF injection at 10 μg/kg/day (or 5 μg/kg/day after chemo-mobilization within 20 days) **or** (b) yielding $<2.0 \times 10^6$ $CD34^+$ cells/kg of body weight in ≥3 apheresis collection; this condition can be challenging from an HPC laboratory standpoint (Olivieri et al. 2012). For such protracted (in days) collections, large quantities of cells have been collected, but the majority of them are not the cells of interest, i.e., most commonly large numbers of granulocytes. Thus, these HPC products require dilution with either autologous plasma or another isotonic solution to a predefined concentration prior to the addition of cryoprotectant and cryopreservation.

From the perspective of the HPC laboratory, cryopreserving and storing cellular products with large volumes involve increased resources as well as increase the risk of adverse events at the time of infusion, namely, cryoprotectant-related toxicities, granulocyte-related reactions, and volume overload (Calmels et al. 2007). Though there is unease that increased TNC concentrations during cryopreservation and storage may result in a higher risk of toxicity to the cells and associated decreased viability, it must once again be mentioned that the ideal TNC cryopreservation concentration has not been identified, and increasing this concentration to achieve smaller product storage volumes is a possibility (Lecchi et al. 2016). Additionally, volume reduction of the HPC product via centrifugation with resulting cell-free supernatant removal could further be utilized to decrease product storage volumes, particularly for those patients that are volume sensitive (i.e., pediatric patients or those with cardiac and/or kidney impairment) or have large-volume products (i.e., from poor mobilizers). These HPC products with smaller volumes would require fewer laboratory materials and reagents, decreased processing time, decreased freezer space, and potentially result in fewer infusion reactions.

4.3.2 Cryopreservation: Storing HPC Products for Later Use

If HPC products cannot be immediately utilized, cryopreservation can be used to preserve the mononuclear cells and maintain their viability and functionality until recipients are ready to receive them (Rowley et al. 1994). In HPC laboratories that have protocols for cryopreservation, this manipulation has been proven to be safe, minimizes adverse events, and allows for timely engraftment of the cells upon later infusion (Koepsell et al. 2014). It is important to note, however, that multiple cryopreservation protocols exist and that each laboratory is tasked with demonstrating that their specific protocols allow for the freezing, storage, thawing, and infusion of viable and functional cells (Lecchi et al. 2016).

While cryopreservation provides many benefits, most notably providing additional time to prepare a patient for transplantation, there are significant risks associated with this process that must be accounted for by the HPC laboratory. Infusion of cryopreserved HPC products is associated with toxicities of variable severity that are related to the total cellular content, cellular composition (i.e., increased number of granulocytes), cryopreservation volume, and overall total product volume (Rich and Cushing 2013). In order to cryopreserve any product, a cryoprotectant must be used in order to prevent the formation of ice crystals within and outside of cells during the freezing process. These ice crystals can result in cell injury/death, decreased viability, and associated complications in recipients. For these reasons, the amount and timing of adding cryoprotectant to HPC products are critical parts of any cryopreservation protocol. Dimethyl sulfoxide (DMSO) is a commonly utilized cryoprotectant, and its use in conjunction with albumin, electrolyte solution, and controlled-rate freezing has been demonstrated to make cryopreservation a safe and effective maneuver in the HPC laboratory. However, it should be noted that laboratories vary in their concentration of cryoprotectant; for DMSO, a commonly used concentration is 10%, but this may be different depending on a particular laboratory's policies, practices, and experience with alternatives (Pamphilon and Mijovic 2007).

4.3.3 Controlled-Rate Freezing Versus Uncontrolled-Rate Freezing

If an HPC product requires cryopreservation, a precise quantity of cryoprotectant is slowly added to a specific number of cells and volume, followed by freezing and subsequent storage in liquid nitrogen (LN2). The process of the actual freezing of an HPC product can transpire in one of two ways: controlled-rate freezing **or** uncontrolled freezing (i.e., dump freezing):

- In controlled-rate freezing, an HPC product is placed within a sealed chamber and cooled at a rate determined by a computer that incorporates temperature data from the product and freezer in real time (often 1–2 °C/min). An important advantage to using controlled-rate freezing is the capacity to minimize the latent heat of fusion phase (see Chap. 6). When the HPC product begins to phase shift during cooling and transitions from a liquid to a solid, energy is released that disrupts the otherwise stable cooling process; this energy is referred to as the latent heat of fusion, and it can result in the temporary warming of cells that may impact cell viability (Meagher and Herzig 1993). With controlled-rate freezing, the temperature of the HPC product is continually measured, and the increasing temperature due to the latent heat of fusion is detected by the computer and is accommodated for by temporarily increasing the rate of cooling until a stable cooling curve is re-achieved. Ultimately, the temperature of the product is decreased to −80 °C or lower prior to transfer to an LN2 storage freezer. During this entire process, the temperature of the product is monitored and recorded.
- In contrast, uncontrolled-rate freezing involves the simple transfer of a HPC product into a −80 °C freezer and subsequently to a LN2 storage freezer (<−150 °C). This process also cools at a general rate of 1–2 °C/min but does not have a mechanism to detect and precisely accommodate for the latent heat of fusion. The actual cooling rate is difficult to document, and the freezer should be left undisturbed, which can be a potential logistical problem for facilities with multiple HPC products to process each day.

In many HPC laboratories, controlled-rate freezing is the choice for cryopreservation of cellular products.

4.3.4 Vapor Phase Liquid Nitrogen Versus Liquid Phase Liquid Nitrogen

At a temperature of −80 °C or lower, a HPC product can be transferred to a LN2 freezer for long-term storage. There are two freezer options for long-term storage of cryopreserved products: vapor phase or liquid phase LN2. Traditionally, liquid phase freezers were known to maintain cell therapy products with fewer temperature fluctuations compared to vapor phase models. However, newer jacketed vapor phase freezers have shown to minimize temperature gradients on par with liquid

Table 4.1 Temperatures for HPC product storage and transport

Product storage	HPC, Apheresis	HPC, Marrow
Fresh HPC product	Room temperature or 1–6 °C up to 72 h	Room temperature up to 48 h[a]
Frozen HPC product in vapor phase LN2	≤−150 °C	≤−150 °C
Frozen HPC product in liquid phase LN2	−196 °C	−196 °C

LN2 liquid nitrogen
[a]Specific facilities may store for longer periods of time and/or at 1–6 °C

phase freezers. Another important benefit of vapor phase LN2 freezers over liquid phase LN2 models is the abrogation of risk associated with viral and bacterial cross-contamination between HPC products housed within the same freezer. In other words, the probability of a potential infectious agent within a cryopreserved cell therapy product contaminating adjacent HPC units is practically zero if storage is conducted in freezers with a gaseous medium versus a liquid medium. There is currently no defined expiration of cryopreserved HPC products, and components frozen for over 10 years old have been successfully thawed and infused with no engraftment issues (see Chap. 6) (Attarian et al. 1996; Veeraputhiran et al. 2010; Winter et al. 2014). See Table 4.1 for temperatures associated with HPC products.

4.3.5 HPC Product Thawing: Fast as You Can

Once the time of transplantation is set, many facilities will thaw a recipient's cryopreserved HPC products as close as possible to the planned infusion time. This is done to minimize the amount of time cells that are retained in the liquid state after thawing prior to infusion. Since some studies have demonstrated that DMSO is cytotoxic to cells at room temperature, rapid thawing in a 37 °C water bath followed by infusion as quickly and safely as possible is recommended (Cameron et al. 2013). While local hospital and laboratory policies must be followed for recipients with multiple products to be infused at a given time, many facilities thaw products sequentially for a given infusion; in this way, confirmation that the antecedent product has been infused successfully and that the recipient is doing well is obtained by the laboratory team from the clinical team prior to thawing of the subsequent HPC product.

4.3.6 DMSO Adverse Effects and Prevention: Taking the Bad with the Good

While the cryoprotectant DMSO has allowed for the effective freezing, storage, and successful transplantation of HPC products, it is also associated with many clinically significant side effects that include nausea, vomiting, cardiovascular events, respiratory distress, kidney injury, and allergic reactions (Tormey and Snyder 2009). Rare fatalities associated with DMSO have even been reported (Zenhausern et al. 2000). In consideration of the documented adverse effects attributed to DMSO, a maximum exposure of 1 g/kg/day is allowed. Depending on the number of TNC collected, the HPC product cell concentration in each bag, product volume, and the weight of the recipient, infusions of HPC products may have to be performed over more than 1 day in order to prevent DMSO-associated toxicities. Due to the medical and logistical challenges associated with DMSO, alternative approaches utilizing decreased concentrations of DMSO (typically 5%) in addition to extracellular protectants like hydroxyethyl starch (HES) have been successful in cryopreserving HPC products. For example, initial data demonstrate improved viability with HES (3%) and DMSO (5%) versus DMSO (10%) alone (Berz et al. 2007). However, there is concern about the use of such solution combinations as there is a paucity of long-term data regarding products cryopreserved in this fashion. Although HES can be a valuable supplement to DMSO that can possibly decrease cryoprotectant-associated adverse events while maintaining or improving cryopreserved HPC product characteristics, the optimal ratio of these agents has not been defined, and the use of such alternatives requires further investigation.

4.3.7 HPC Product Washing: To Wash or Not to Wash?

Due to the adverse events known to be associated with cryoprotectants such as DMSO, it is logical to consider the option of washing HPC products after thawing in order to remove the offending chemical. However, washing of the cells to remove DMSO and other additives risks loss of critical HPCs due to cytotoxicity associated with increased exposure time of cells to DMSO as well as HPC losses that would occur during washing process; both of these would result in a lowering of the cell dose. In selected circumstances, such as in patients with a documented severe DMSO allergy, washing of HPC products may be the safer choice. But as a matter of routine practice, it is more common to infuse the HPC product directly into the patient after the thawing process is completed.

4.4 Allogeneic Products: Unique Concerns and Unique Processes

In contrast to autologous HPC products, allogeneic HPC products harbor attendant risks just as any routine blood component from the blood bank. These risks include, but are not limited to, infectious disease transmission, allergic reactions, immunologic reactions, hemolytic reactions, and graft-versus-host disease. Additionally, unlike in solid organ allografts, transplantation across ABO barriers with HPC components is routinely performed. However, the many donor and product factors which might make a routine blood donor and corresponding product ineligible and

Table 4.2 ABO mismatches in HPC allogeneic transplantation

	O donor	A donor	B donor	AB donor
O recipient	Compatible	Major	Major	Major
A recipient	Minor	Compatible	Major and minor	Major
B recipient	Minor	Major and minor	Compatible	Major
AB recipient	Minor	Minor	Minor	Compatible

unsuitable for donation or transfusion may not automatically exclude the same individual for donation of HPC products. In contrast to donors of routine blood components, the potentially detrimental factors associated with an HPC donor and corresponding product are weighed against the benefit of transplantation of the impacted HPC product for a given recipient on a case-by-case basis.

A donor-recipient pair is considered to have a major ABO mismatch if the recipient's plasma has naturally occurring isohemagglutinins that are incompatible with the donor's red cells (e.g., A donor and O recipient). Conversely, the donor-recipient pair is considered to have a minor ABO mismatch if the donor's plasma contains naturally occurring isohemagglutinins against the recipient's red cells (e.g., O donor and B recipient). Certain donor-recipient pairs can have both major and minor (also termed bidirection) ABO mismatches (e.g., A donor and B recipient). See Table 4.2 for a complete presentation of ABO mismatches between donors and recipients.

4.4.1 HPC, Apheresis Allogeneic Products and ABO Incompatibility

HPC, Apheresis products collected from the peripheral blood usually have hematocrits <5%; thus, issues of major ABO incompatibility due to incompatible red cells rarely occur. The apheresis instruments are excellent at isolating the buffy coat and limiting the red cell contamination of the HPC product. On the other hand, these products can have up to several hundred milliliters of plasma, and thus possible hemolytic reaction due to incompatible isohemagglutinins can occur. This may necessitate plasma reduction as part of the HPC processing. See Tables 4.2 and 4.3 for complete information on donor-recipient ABO mismatches and associated HPC laboratory processes to mitigate the risk of acute reactions. FACT/JACIE Standards require that the transplant physician specify the modifications that should occur to the HPC product based on the ABO incompatibilities present between the donor and recipient (Foundation for the Accreditation of Cellular Therapy, Joint Accreditation Committee-ISCT and EBMT 2015).

For HPC, Apheresis products that have incompatible isohemagglutinins against recipient red cells (i.e., minor ABO incompatibility), plasma reduction to remove the isohemagglutinins can be achieved by centrifugal separation. This can be performed by either manual centrifugation of the product bag and expressing off excess plasma or by using an automated apheresis instrument to remove plasma. However,

Table 4.3 Required HPC product modifications based on ABO mismatches

Donor	Recipient	Manipulation to the product
O	O	None
O	A, B, AB	Plasma reduction
A	A	None
A	O	Red cell reduction
A	B	Red cell and plasma reduction
A	AB	Plasma reduction
B	B	None
B	A	Red cell and plasma reduction
B	O	Red cell reduction
B	AB	Plasma reduction
AB	AB	None
AB	O, A, B	Red cell reduction

Red cell reductions are routinely performed on HPC, Marrow products only. Plasma reductions are routinely performed on HPC, Apheresis and HPC, Marrow products

the benefits of plasma reduction must be weighed against the risk of cell losses that may occur during the separation.

HPC, Apheresis products may be infused either fresh or after cryopreservation and subsequent thawing. If cryopreservation is applied, the identical methods previously discussed for autologous HPC products can be utilized.

4.4.2 HPC, Marrow Allogeneic Products and ABO Incompatibility

HPC, Marrow products collected from anesthetized donors in the operative suite can routinely have volumes of up to 2000 ml with hematocrits of up to 35%; thus, hemolytic reactions due to incompatible donor red cells can occur. Most facilities determine their own maximum limit for the allowable quantity of incompatible red cells, with 20–30 ml of incompatible red cells being regarded as acceptable (Daniel-Johnson and Schwartz 2011). However, if this threshold is exceeded, red cell reduction must be performed.

All methodologies for red cell reduction are based upon densitometric separation of red cells with a specific gravity of approximately 1.08–1.09 from MNCs with a similar specific gravity of approximately 1.06–1.07 (Areman and Loper 2016). These methods include procedures previously discussed such as centrifugation and automated apheresis separation, as well as two additional methods: hydroxyethyl starch-mediated densitometric separation and densitometric gradient separation. When red cells come into contact with the hydroxyethyl starch, red cell rouleaux occur, and the specific gravity of the red cell fraction increases. This results in a better densitometric separation between the sedimenting red cells and the mononuclear cells that remain afloat. The red cells can then be removed, leaving behind a MNC-enriched product.

Densitometric gradient separations utilize agents, such as Hypaque-Ficoll, to create a density barrier. Red cells and granulocytes have a higher specific gravity and, after a centrifugation step, end up below the density gradient barrier. Cellular elements with a lower specific gravity, such as the mononuclear cells containing the cells of interest, remain above the gradient and can be subsequently isolated. Similar to plasma reduction, the benefits of any red cell reduction strategy versus the risks of HPC losses must be considered.

Additionally, HPC, Marrow products also contain large quantities of plasma. If a minor ABO incompatibility exists between the donor and recipient, the product would require a plasma reduction, as described previously.

HPC, Marrow products may be infused either fresh or after cryopreservation and subsequent thawing. If cryopreservation is applied, the identical methods previously discussed for autologous HPC products can be utilized. HPC, Marrow products undergo red cell reduction prior to cryopreservation to minimize hemolysis and the deleterious effects of free hemoglobin (Rother et al. 2005).

4.4.3 Donor Lymphocyte Infusion: Small Infusions for Big Issues

In cases of allogeneic HPC transplantation where recipients have disease relapse or there is evidence of failing engraftment (e.g., worsening chimerism studies), few treatment options are available short of a second allogeneic transplant. In these situations, donor lymphocyte infusion (DLI) may be considered to re-induce remission by eliciting a graft-versus-tumor effect and/or to provide support to a failing graft in the hopes of improvement. The exact concentrations and frequency of DLI can vary from patient to patient and from disease to disease. Often DLI dosing is utilized to achieve a specific improvement endpoint or until adverse events manifest (graft-versus-host disease or marrow toxicity) (Castagna et al. 2016).

For the HPC laboratory, DLI is processed from one of two sources: either from the original allogeneic HPC product prior to transplantation or from a subsequent leukocyte collection at a later time after transplantation from the original allogeneic donor. When processing DLI for potential future use from the original allogeneic HPC product, the $CD3^+$ cells need to be quantified and cryopreserved for use at a later time. $CD3^+$ cells are most commonly enumerated and dosed per kg of recipient body weight. The volumes of DLI are much smaller than typical HPC transplant volumes. However, it should be noted that $CD3^+$ cell populations are not necessarily directly proportional to $CD34^+$ cell populations; thus, depending on the dose(s) of DLI requested by the transplant physician and the $CD34^+$ dose requested, clear communication should be provided to the clinical team taking care of the recipient so that the updated $CD34^+$ cell dose, reduced as a result of any requested DLI processing and storage, is known and verified as this may alter the original request for DLI doses. After preparation of DLI at requested doses, these aliquots of cells are cryopreserved per standard protocols as described above and are thawed and infused similar to traditional HPC products. DLI processed from a subsequent collection from an allogeneic donor is similarly enumerated, processed, cryopreserved, stored, thawed, and infused. However, the majority of DLIs are provided fresh. Donor collection volumes are proportional to T-cell collection and thus can be tailored to the requested dose. The donor must be reevaluated prior to each new collection to ensure safety of the product and the donation.

4.5 Infectious Disease Testing: Impact on the HPC Laboratory

While an in-depth discussion of infectious disease testing for HPC donors is covered elsewhere in this volume, it is important to highlight the impact that results of these tests have on the HPC laboratory. Testing for infectious disease agents must be performed per manufacturer's instructions using FDA-licensed and FDA-approved donor screening tests. While testing is not required for autologous donors, any untested products must be labeled as "Not Evaluated For Infectious Substances" and stored in quarantine vapor phase LN2 freezers. Additionally, for any donor (either autologous or allogeneic) that has an "incomplete" or "ineligible" status based on the results of the donor screening questions and/or testing, the corresponding product must have the appropriate labeling and be stored in quarantine vapor phase LN2 freezers.

As stated previously, some allogeneic donors may not meet all donation requirements but may still be approved for donation. In these situations, a summary of records that contains information regarding why those requirements have not been met must be provided to the transplant center prior to product procurement. The recipient's physician has the ability to authorize the use of the product if the recipient has been advised and the product is labeled appropriately and released under urgent medical need. Clear and timely communication between the transplant physicians (for both donor and recipient) and the HPC laboratory is critical to ensure the appropriate labeling, processing, storage, and handling of such HPC products.

4.6 Potency of the HPC Product

Regulatory and accrediting standards of HPC laboratories require processes and protocols to confirm product identity, trace the product from donor to recipient, and characterize product integrity for quality and quantity. For each institution, release criteria are established for donor eligibility, total cell count, HPC cell dose, viability, and sterility, and acceptable values and ranges must be defined. There is a need for some variability in what is "acceptable" as these products, which are derived from and for individuals, are potentially irreplaceable and needed urgently. With regard to viability, post-processing (pre-cryopreservation) TNC viability release criteria is typically >90%, with post-thaw viabilities having a lower threshold of >70%. The equipment, reagents, and supplies used in all HPC laboratory processes must be qualified, written definitions of the type and volume of samples to be obtained must be stated, and time points during production for sampling must be determined. It should be clearly defined whether quality control is an in-process control or whether it is a control of the final product. Even minor manipulations, such as wash steps, volume reduction steps, and cryopreservation, require quality testing for cell numbers and bacterial and fungal contamination. Autologous and allogeneic HPC products have a well-established and proven clinical benefit for patients, and these unique products can be released despite quality control parameters being out of specification. The final decision to release an HPC product that does not meet specifications should be guided by the consideration that the benefits outweigh potential risks for the recipient. Lastly, any adverse events that occur during or after HPC infusion that might be related to the product should be documented and reported to the HPC laboratory. Only with this information can processes be improved, errors identified and corrected, and products ultimately made safer and better for patients.

4.6.1 Product Release Testing

Testing requirements for the release of cellular therapy products must be defined. Product testing and characterization ensure product safety, purity, and potency, but currently no standardization exists for what to test, when to test, and how to test HPC and other cellular therapy products. Additionally, the combination of manual and automated methods commonly employed further contributes to the variability observed between different facilities. Commonly performed tests include TNC count, hematocrit, viability, sterility, $CD34^+$ cell content for HPC products, and T-cell content for allogeneic products. These tests may also play a role in determining processing procedures, such as RBC removal, MNC and/or subset enrichment, or depletion of other target cells. Protocols for test utilization are established with consideration of timing for each particular manipulation in the overall processing of a product. For example, determination of $CD34^+$ cell content both before and after density gradient separation is performed, as this process is known to decrease $CD34^+$ cell content.

TNC and $CD34^+$ counts are general measures of product quantity but do not provide information about viability or potency. Commonly used viability assays include flow cytometry-based assays and dye exclusion assays. The use of 7-aminoactinomycin D (7-AAD), a fluorescent chemical compound with DNA affinity, in flow cytometric analyses offers advantages over traditional trypan blue staining that include decreased subjectivity, increased accuracy (particularly with thawed HPC products), and the ability to be done in conjunction with $CD34^+$ assessment. However, depending on the processing laboratory setup, turnaround times for flow-based assays may hinder the lab's ability to release a product for fresh infusion; in this circumstance, the use of trypan blue can be advantageous.

Potency assays are performed to assess the ability of a specific cellular therapy product to affect a specific result, the most common example being the use of a hematopoietic progenitor cell transplant to result in marrow reconstitution. These assays have been found to be associated with time to engraftment (Stroncek et al. 2007) Examples of these include TNC count, CD34$^+$ assessment, colony-forming unit assays, and measurement of CD133$^+$/aldehyde dehydrogenase (ALDH) bright cells. Emerging methods include gene and microRNA expression profiling.

Finally, assessments of sterility are performed to query the product for aerobic and anaerobic bacteria and fungus. Culture-based methods are the most common in US labs and require validation by each processing center for the products and reagents used. Other rapid methods are needed for more than minimally manipulated products and may include gram staining, endotoxin measurement, and mycoplasma testing.

Additional considerations for release testing include labeling and assessment of product appearance (e.g., color, turbidity, and container integrity). Cell composition, storage conditions, product expiration, patient identification, product identification, processing center name and address, warnings, and precautions are common release requirements. The implementation of ISBT labeling has helped to move standardization forward in this matter (Slaper-Cortenbach 2010).

4.7 Expert Point of View

HPC transplantation, whether autologous or allogeneic, is a routine treatment in many institutions. The HPC laboratory plays a critical role in guaranteeing the safety and efficacy of these products regardless of whether they are immediately infused or cryopreserved and stored for years prior to use (Koepsell et al. 2014). There are many things about HPC product processing that are defined and required. However, some issues that can impact patient safety or efficacy are not well defined and/or vary from facility to facility.

For autologous HPC product processing, the optimal concentration of TNC in the HPC products prior to cryopreservation is unknown. Autologous HPC products are almost always cryopreserved, and DMSO is the most commonly used cryopreservation agent at this time (we currently use a 10% concentration). Cell concentration in HPC product bags and the percent DMSO used in cryopreservation are two laboratory variables that have direct impacts on how much DMSO a patient will receive at the time of transplant (Windrum et al. 2005). Autologous donors with high peripheral white blood cell counts and low circulating CD34$^+$ counts (i.e., poor mobilizers) can have large volumes of product collected, processed, and stored, which can lead to large-volume infusions at the time of transplantation. These transplants often require infusion over multiple days to ensure patient safety and limit adverse side effects related to the cryoprotectant as well as cellular content. Some institutions have even limited the daily DMSO dose of cryopreserved products to decrease infusion-related adverse events (Khera et al. 2012). Regardless of the freezing method, HPC products are carefully cryopreserved to maintain cellular viability and functionality. Cell viability is critical to engraftment of transplanted HPCs; therefore, the time from addition of cryopreservation media to start of controlled-rate freezing (our preferred option) must be minimized, as DMSO is cytotoxic to cells when in the liquid state (Rowley and Anderson 1993). Regulatory and accrediting agencies require the validation and monitoring of a cryopreservation method and storage that preserves cellular viability both post-processing (pre-cryopreservation) and at infusion (post-thaw). Post-processing (pre-cryopreservation) TNC viability release criteria is typically >90%, with post-thaw viabilities typically at lower levels of >70%.

Unlike autologous HPCs, allogeneic HPCs may be ABO incompatible. If a donor-recipient ABO incompatibility exists, the ordering stem cell transplantation team member must indicate the type of ABO incompatibility, and if RBC reduction is needed for the removal of incompatible RBCs (our recommended threshold is <20 ml), plasma reduction is needed to remove incompatible plasma or both in the donor HPC product. Similarly, DLI doses to be prepared and cryopreserved must be requested, with the understanding that if these cells are to be taken from the original HPC product, a smaller $CD34^+$ transplantable dose will be an obligatory effect.

4.8 Future Directions

There are many unanswered questions in the area of HPC processing. We still do not know the optimal TNC concentration prior to cryopreservation. This, of course, may be impacted by the concentration and/or type of cryoprotectant utilized. While 10% DMSO is currently the most common cryopreservative in use, lower concentrations of DMSO in conjunction with other agents (such as hydroxyethyl starch) could decrease recipient exposure to this chemical associated with a variety of adverse events (Windrum et al. 2005). However, long-term stability data of cryopreserved HPCs in predefined and optimized alternative solutions are needed. Lastly, adverse event monitoring, which might be considered a clinical problem, has direct connections with the HPC laboratory. Through the reporting, tracking, and reviewing of adverse events via a robust quality program that monitors adverse events and associates them with HPC laboratory variables, a safer and more effective HPC laboratory and overall program can be created.

References

Areman EM, Loper K (2016) Cellular therapy: principles, methods, and regulations, 2nd edn. AABB Press, Bethesda, MD

Attarian H, Feng Z, Buckner CD, MacLeod B, Rowley SD (1996) Long-term cryopreservation of bone marrow for autologous transplantation. Bone Marrow Transplant 17:425–430

Berz D, McCormack EM, Winer ES, Colvin GA, Quesenberry PJ (2007) Cryopreservation of hematopoietic stem cells. Am J Hematol 82:463–472

Calmels B, Lemarie C, Esterni B et al (2007) Occurrence and severity of adverse events after autologous hematopoietic progenitor cell infusion are related to the amount of granulocytes in the apheresis product. Transfusion 47:1268–1275

Cameron G, Filer K, Hall A, Hogge D (2013) Evaluation of post-thaw blood progenitor product integrity and viability over time at room temperature and 4C. Cytotherapy 15:S27

Castagna L, Sarina B, Bramanti S, Perseghin P, Mariotti J, Morabito L (2016) Donor lymphocyte infusion after allogeneic stem cell transplantation. Transfus Apher Sci 54:345–355

Daniel-Johnson J, Schwartz J (2011) How do I approach ABO-incompatible hematopoietic progenitor cell transplantation? Transfusion 51:1143–1149

Foundation for the Accreditation of Cellular Therapy, Joint Accreditation Committee-ISCT and EBMT (2015) FACT-JACIE international standards for hematopoietic cellular therapy product collection, processing, and administration, 6th edn. The Foundation for the Accreditation of Cellular Therapy, Omaha, NE

Khera N, Jinneman J, Storer BE et al (2012) Limiting the daily total nucleated cell dose of cryopreserved peripheral blood stem cell products for autologous transplantation improves infusion-related safety with no adverse impact on hematopoietic engraftment. Biol Blood Marrow Transplant 18:220–228

Koepsell SA, Jacob EK, McKenna DH (2014) The collection and processing of hematopoietic stem cells. In: Fung MK, Grossman BJ, Hillyer CD, Westhoff CM (eds) Technical manual, 18th edn. AABB Press, Bethesda, MD

Lecchi L, Giovanelli S, Gagliardi B, Pezzali I, Ratti I, Marconi M (2016) An update on methods for cryopreservation and thawing of hematopoietic stem cells. Transfus Apher Sci 54:324–336

Meagher RC, Herzig RH (1993) Techniques of harvesting and cryopreservation of stem cells. Hematol Oncol Clin North Am 7:501–533

Olivieri A, Marchetti M, Lemoli R et al (2012) Proposed definition of 'poor mobilizer' in lymphoma and multiple myeloma: an analytic hierarchy process by ad hoc working group Gruppo ItalianoTrapianto di Midollo Osseo. Bone Marrow Transplant 47:342–351

Pamphilon D, Mijovic A (2007) Storage of hematopoietic stem cells. Asian J Transfus Sci 1:71–76

Rich A, Cushing MM (2013) Adverse events associated with hematopoietic progenitor cell product infusion. In: Shaz BH, Hillyer CD, Roshal M, Abrams CS (eds) Transfusion medicine and hemostasis: clinical and laboratory aspects, 2nd edn. Elsevier Inc., Amsterdam

Rother RP, Bell L, Hillmen P, Gladwin MT (2005) The clinical sequelae of intravascular hemolysis and extracellular plasma hemoglobin: a novel mechanism of human disease. JAMA 293:1653–1662

Rowley SD, Anderson GL (1993) Effect of DMSO exposure without cryopreservation on hematopoietic progenitor cells. Bone Marrow Transplant 11:389–393

Rowley SD, Bensinger WI, Gooley TA, Buckner CD (1994) Effect of cell concentration on bone marrow and peripheral blood stem cell cryopreservation. Blood 83:2731–2736

Slaper-Cortenbach I (2010) ISBT 128 coding and labeling for cellular therapy products. Cell Tissue Bank 11:375–378

Stroncek DF, Jin P, Wang E, Jett B (2007) Potency analysis of cellular therapies: the emerging role of molecular assays. J Transl Med 5:24

Tormey CA, Snyder EL (2009) Transfusion support for the oncology patient. In: Simon TL, Snyder EL, Solheim BG, Stowell CP, Strauss RG, Petrides M (eds) Rossi's principles of transfusion medicine, 4th edn. Blackwell Publishing Ltd, West Sussex

Veeraputhiran M, Theus JW, Pesek G, Barlogie B, Cottler-Fox M (2010) Viability and engraftment of hematopoietic progenitor cells after long-term cryopreservation: effect of diagnosis and percentage dimethyl sulfoxide concentration. Cytotherapy 12(6):764

Windrum P, Morris TC, Drake MB, Niederwieser D, Ruutu T, Chronic Leukaemia EBMT (2005) Working party complications subcommittee. Variation in dimethyl sulfoxide use in stem cell transplantation: a survey of EBMT centres. Bone Marrow Transplant 36:601–603

Winter JM, Jacobson P, Bullough B, Christensen AP, Boyer M, Reems JA (2014) Long-term effects of cryopreservation on clinically prepared hematopoietic progenitor cell products. Cytotherapy 16:965–975

Zenhausern R, Tobler A, Leoncini L, Hess OM, Ferrari P (2000) Fatal cardiac arrhythmia after infusion of dimethyl sulfoxide-cryopreserved hematopoietic stem cells in a patient with severe primary cardiac amyloidosis and end-stage renal failure. Ann Hematol 79:523–526

CD34+ Enrichment and T-Cell Depletion

5

Scott T. Avecilla and Cheryl A. Goss

5.1 Introduction

Hematopoietic progenitor cells (HPCs) are collected from various sources which include bone marrow aspiration, apheresis collection from cytokine-mobilized donors, as well as umbilical cord blood. These grafts are heterogenous in their composition in that they include HPCs, myeloid lineage cells, lymphoid lineage cells (T cells and B cells), red blood cells, and platelets. Some constituents such as CD3+ T cells of the grafts have been implicated in the serious complication of graft-versus-host disease (G*v*HD), a condition wherein the donor immune cells recognize the recipient as nonself and results in attack of recipient tissues. While there have been major advances in the understanding of immunity and its regulation and thus avenues to pharmacologically modulate the immune response, our ability to mitigate unwanted alloreactivity is thus far incomplete. With the emerging understanding of which cellular subsets are important to hematopoietic reconstitution comes the ability to engineer HPC grafts to influence their biological characteristics. One effective method to engineer HPC grafts has been to use specific cellular markers to enrich or deplete a graft of target cells in a process called immunomagnetic cell selection.

S.T. Avecilla, M.D., Ph.D. (✉)
Cell Therapy Laboratory Services, Department of Laboratory Medicine, Memorial Sloan Kettering Cancer Center, New York, NY, USA
e-mail: avecills@mskcc.org

C.A. Goss, M.D.
Transfusion Medicine Service Department of Laboratory Medicine, Memorial Sloan Kettering Cancer Center, New York, NY, USA
e-mail: gossc@mskcc.org

J. Schwartz, B.H. Shaz (eds.), *Best Practices in Processing and Storage for Hematopoietic Cell Transplantation*, Advances and Controversies in Hematopoietic Transplantation and Cell Therapy,
https://doi.org/10.1007/978-3-319-58949-7_5

5.2 Methods of Cell Selection

The foundation of cell selection firmly rests on the principle that specific proteins are expressed, often uniquely, on the surface of cells which identify their level of differentiation and functional characteristics. The most widely adopted technique of cell selection utilizes monoclonal antibodies targeted to specific cluster of differentiation (CD) to mark the cells of interest. By coupling the monoclonal antibodies to a "hooking" mechanism, the target cells can be separated from complex cellular mixtures with ease at clinically relevant scales. Two major selection strategies exist, and they are called positive selection and negative selection.

5.2.1 Positive Selection for CD34$^+$ Cells

The aim for *positive cell selection* strategies is to mark and capture the target cell of interest for use as the HPC graft. In the case of *CD34$^+$ positive cell selection* or CD34$^+$ enrichment, a paramagnetically labeled CD34 monoclonal antibody reagent is mixed with the HPC, Apheresis (HPC(A)) product to first tag the cells. After washing off unbound antibody, the cell suspension is passed through a column of strong magnetic field. Due to magnetic flux effects of the column, the CD34$^+$ cells are retained in the column, while unlabeled cells pass through as the bypass fraction. Once all the cell suspension has been applied to the column and the column has been washed to ensure that only the CD34$^+$ cells are retained, the magnetic field is withdrawn, and the cells are eluted off the column and used as the HPC product (Fig. 5.1a). The major steps of this procedure and some points of procedure troubleshooting are presented in Tables 5.1 and 5.2. This strategy is very effective at enriching the product for CD34$^+$ cells with purities of 90–99% commonly obtained. In this case, the HPCs have been separated from all the other cellular constituents of the original product, and thereby it is a method for passive T-cell reduction or depletion. Since CD34$^+$ is the most widely accepted marker for progenitor content in HPC products, it was logical that this strategy was first employed. Target cell recovery has been reported to be 50–100% when successfully performed (Keever-Taylor et al. 2012) and a passive CD3$^+$ T-cell reduction of greater than 3-log.

5.2.2 Negative Selection (T Cell Depletion)

In *negative selection* procedures, the target cell population(s) is undesirable and is actively removed from the HPC product (Fig. 5.1b). One of the earliest *negative selection* methods used CD3$^+$/19$^+$ cells as the target which resulted in HPC products with extremely low levels of residual CD3$^+$/19$^+$ cells. One drawback to this strategy is that there was an increase of graft rejection/failure. In order to reduce the incidence of this rejection, some investigators supplement the HPC graft by adding back a fixed dose of CD3$^+$/19$^+$ cells (Geyer et al. 2012). One major benefit to

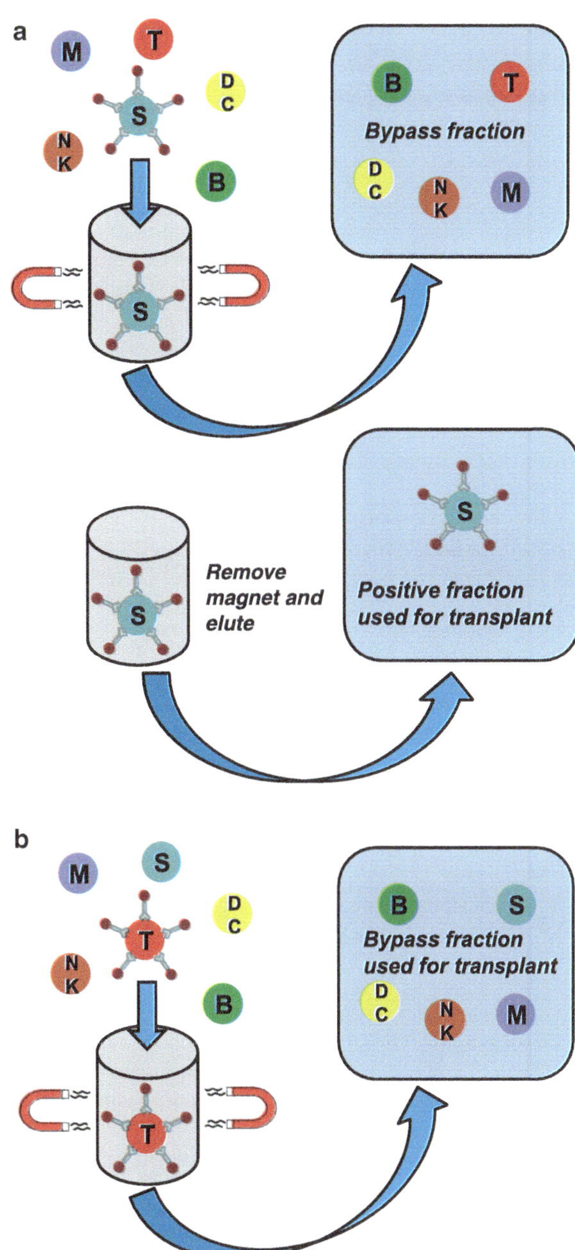

Fig. 5.1 Cell selection schema. (**a**) Positive cell selection schema: a heterogenous mixture of hematopoietic cells is mixed with a magnetically labeled monoclonal antibody targeting the cell type of interest to be enriched. The labeled cell mixture is then passed through a ferromagnetic column to retain the target cell and remove the nontarget cell populations (bypass fraction). The magnetic field is removed from the column, and the target cell population ($CD34^+$ cell) can be eluted for use. (**b**) Negative cell selection schema: similar to positive selection, a heterogenous mixture of hematopoietic cells is mixed with a magnetically labeled monoclonal antibody targeting the cell type of interest to be removed. In contrast to positive selection, however, the cells that bypass the column contain the desired cell populations ($CD34^+$ cells, NKs, etc.), while the cells retained in the column are discarded. *S* $CD34^+$ cells, *T* T cells, *B* B cells, *M* macrophages/monocytes, *NK* natural killer, *DC* dendritic cells

negative selection is the retention of other cell populations such as natural killer (NK) cells in the HPC graft which could aid in providing an antitumor effect. Newer targets for *negative "specific" selection* include T-cell receptor (TcR) α/β (Aversa 2015) and $CD45RA^+$ cells (Teschner et al. 2014) (discussed next).

Table 5.1 CD34⁺ cell selection workflow example

Selection processing steps	Process
1. Preselection sampling/ testing	(a) Flow cytometry (CD34, CD3 with subsets) (b) 5-day sterility (Bactec bottles) (c) Hematology (WBC, HCT, PLT, DIFF) (d) ABO/Rh confirmation
2. Preprocessing HPC product storage	Products are diluted with a human serum albumin buffer or other compatible solution to a cell concentration of <200 × 10E6 ml whenever possible
3. Platelet removal	Perform two (2) platelet washes to remove the majority of platelets
4. Human IVIG	Human IVIG may be added to the washed product and incubated for 5 min at room temperature to reduce nonspecific binding of the target antibody during the incubation step
5. Post-incubation wash step	Wash product once to remove any excess unbound antibody
6. Product resuspension and examination	Resuspend product to the appropriate volume for loading on the machine, and process according to manufacturer's instructions
7. Concentration of final $CD34^+$ selected cell fraction	At completion of $CD34^+$ selection procedure, transfer $CD34^+$ cell fraction to four 50 mL conical centrifuge tubes. Spin tubes for 10 min (730 × *g*), resuspend washed cell pellet, and pool into one tube at a predetermined volume
8. Post-selection tests	(a) Flow cytometry (CD34, CD3 with subsets) (b) LAL endotoxin (c) 14-day sterility (d) Stat Gram stain (e) CFU (where applicable) (f) Nucleated cell count (TNC)

Table 5.2 Potential problems and troubleshooting

Issue	Solution
Platelet clumping preprocessing	Perform two (2) platelet washes to remove the majority of platelets. Excess platelet contamination causes product clumping which can interfere with successful cell selection and cell recovery
Nonspecific binding of target antibody (e.g., CD34)	Human IVIG may be added to the washed product and incubated for 5 min at room temperature (optional)
Clumping during product resuspension (post-target-antibody incubation)	Run product through a filter (170–260 μm filter). May require multiple passes/filters to remove all clumps
Product TNC at or exceeds limit for device tubing set (12.0 × 10E10 nucleated cells) [CD34 selection]	Split the product and run over two large-scale columns. Avoid fluidic problems and retain high levels of recovery

5.2.2.1 T-Cell Receptor Specific (Negative) Selection

Studies have shown γ/δ T lymphocytes, in the allogeneic hematopoietic cell transplant (allo-HCT) setting, are beneficial effector cells (Doherty 1992). They have strong antitumor effect, play a role in antimicrobial defense, and usually do not cause GvHD (Lamb et al. 1996; Drobyski et al. 1999). The γ/δ T lymphocytes represent a small portion of the total T-cell population (2–10%), while α/β T lymphocytes predominate (Daniele et al. 2012). New *negative selection* methods targeting the α/β TCR have been developed to remove these lymphocytes from the product while leaving behind the γ/δ T lymphocytes, NK cells, and $CD34^+$ HPCs (Table 5.3). The most commonly employed method uses monoclonal antibodies against the α/β TcR followed by immunomagnetic removal of the targeted α/β T lymphocytes. Of note, due to limitations of the currently available selection reagents and tubing sets for α/β TcR, the total nucleated cell (TNC) that can be processed is effectively 50% less than allowed on the large-scale $CD34^+$ enrichment reagent, currently only able to process 6.0×10^{10} nucleated cells. In contrast to CD34 enrichment where the target cell population is typically 0.5–1.5% of the total cell number, α/β TcR negative selection aims to remove an abundant cell target (20–50% of total cell number). This key difference results in the aforementioned reduced TNC cell capacity that can be accommodated in the processing kit. The implications of reduced cell capacity for the processing is that either less of the collected cells can be processed or that multiple processing events need to be performed to accommodate the entirety of the collection. In the first scenario, the result of processing less of the collected material is that lower CD34 cell doses will result, whereas in the second scenario, the resource utilization would increase two- to threefold which could make the transplant difficult to make available due to financial and labor limitations. The literature indicates that $>2 \times 10^6$ $CD34^+$ cells/kg of recipient body weight is an adequate cell dose for unmodified HPC(A) and HPC(M), and it is likely that such doses may be provided with single-day collection. However, with α/β TcR *negative selections*, there are many transplantation situations, such as large recipients (>90 kg actual body weight) or smaller donors who do not sufficiently mobilize $CD34^+$ cells to yield adequate $CD34^+$ cell doses. When centers consider implementing this relatively new cell selection strategy, it will be important to assess the implications of being able to only process half the previous amount of cells. This may necessitate performing multiple parallel cell selections which can rapidly overwhelm available cell processing laboratory resources. From a regulatory and accrediting standpoint, it should be noted that immunomagnetic cell selection is considered minimal manipulation by the FDA (FDA 2014) because the function of the cells is not altered and the HPC product is still intended for homologous use. From a clinical perspective, minimal manipulation means that the cells will retain their intrinsic capabilities as HPCs; however, by the removal or enrichment of target cell types, the risk of

Table 5.3 Graft cell types and their biological effects

Cell type	Biological effect
$CD34^+$ cells	Hematopoietic reconstitution
$CD3^+$TCRα/β+cells	G*v*HD
$CD3^+$TCRγ/δ+cells	Adoptive immunity; antitumor activity
NK cells	Antitumor activity
$CD45RA^+$ cells	G*v*HD
$CD19^+$ cells	B-cells which may carry risk of Epstein-Barr virus-driven posttransplantation lymphoproliferative disorder

unwanted outcomes such as GvHD can be reduced. Other methods of cell processing that involve growth in culture and/or genetic engineering, which can markedly alter the biological activity of the cells, can be associated with unpredictable biological behaviors which increase the risk of their use in humans. Latter situation is considered more than minimal manipulation which carries a higher amount of scrutiny by accrediting agencies and regulatory inspectors.

5.3 Marrow Selection

The previously presented information on HPC cell selections have focused primarily upon the immunomagnetic selection of HPC, Apheresis products. Due to the fact that HPC(A) has a high white blood cell content relative to red blood cell (RBC) content, with hematocrit (HCT) levels most often below 5%, it has been the most widely used starting material for cell selections since interference from other cellular components such as RBCs is minimal and the product is highly concentrated. Other HPC sources such as bone marrow (HPC(M)) and cord blood (HPC(CB)) require additional manufacturing steps to allow for successful selection. HPC(M) is thought to have a somewhat different composition of cellular constituents which possibly include more primitive HPCs at earlier stages of pluripotency (Theilgaard-Monch et al. 2003). In some cases, HPC(M) may also be the only HPC that is available. Some donors may only wish to donate marrow to avoid being exposed to G-CSF injections for 5 or more days and subsequent apheresis procedures. Additionally, certain donors, such as those with hemoglobinopathies like sickle cell trait, may not qualify to receive G-CSF for donor safety concerns. Typically, HPC(M) has a substantial RBC content with HCT levels up to 30%. Empirical evidence using HPC(A) for cell selections suggested that products with a HCT of greater than 4% was associated with an excessive amount of cell clumping at various stages of cell selection (Avecilla et al. 2016). In order for HPC(M) to successfully undergo CD34$^+$ cell selection, methods to mitigate interference from RBCs must be performed. One method utilizes hydroxyethyl starch (HES) and gravity sedimentation to achieve extensively RBC-reduced HPC(M) product. The RBCs are induced to undergo rouleaux formation and allowed to sediment to the bottom of the product bag. A nucleated cell-rich buffy coat is established at the interface between the RBCs and the supernatant. The buffy coat is subsequently transferred to another bag to separate the target nucleated cells (NCs) from the bulk of the RBCs. The RBC-reduced HPC(M) product then undergoes a washing step to remove the HES, and the product is resuspended in buffer. Once in buffer, the HPC(M) product is processed according to manufacturer's instructions for CD34$^+$ selection. CD34$^+$ enrichment of HPC(M) with the CliniMACS® CD34$^+$ Reagent System (Miltenyi Biotec Inc., San Diego, CA) produces final products that are comparable to HPC(A) in CD34$^+$ cell purity (>70%), viability (>70%), and recovery (>50%). T-cell reduction was also found to be satisfactory (log reduction >3.0). Due to the lower CD34$^+$ cell content of HPC(M) as compared to HPC(A), special consideration has to be given at various steps of processing to ensure adequate cell doses are retained and not lost. Figure 5.2 is an example of a notification and decision tree workflow. By making conservative assumptions of CD34+ cell content and cell recovery at key steps and taking into account the RBC compatibility of the product, the TNC and CD34+ cell content (when available) can be estimated at several points in the process. This allows the procedure to be stopped to ensure adequate cell dose and not proceed to RBC reduction and/or cell selection where additional CD34+ cell losses are expected.

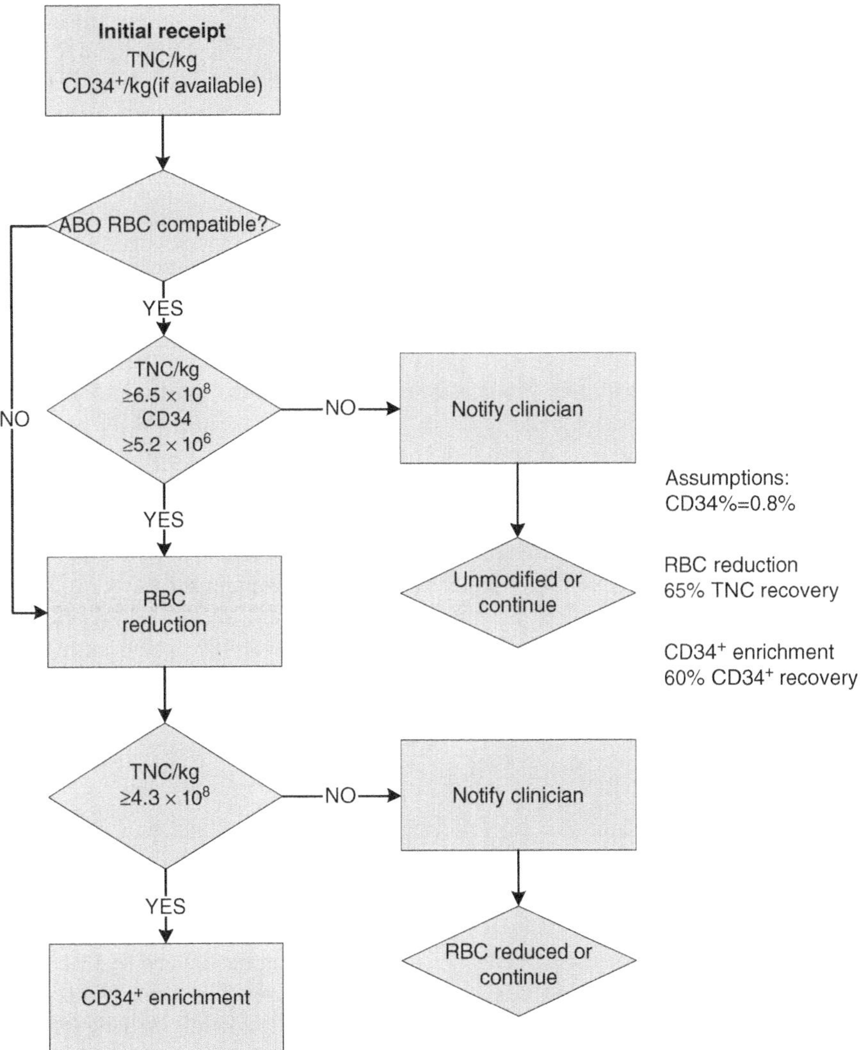

Fig. 5.2 Decision and notification algorithm for CD34+ cell-enriched HPC(M)

5.4 Donor Considerations

Cell selection procedures can result in a substantial target cell loss; therefore, the $CD34^+$ cell content should be as high as possible to ensure the production of an adequate graft. Despite careful donor screening, it is not possible to predict whether an allogeneic donor will mobilize a sufficient number of HPCs with G CSF alone. If multiple days of collection are necessary to collect the target $CD34^+$ cell dose, most laboratories do not have the resources to perform selections for each day. Some transplant groups have begun to use peripheral blood $CD34^+$ cell testing and mobilization augmentation with plerixafor (Hauge et al. 2014; Gattillo et al. 2015; Nadeau et al. 2015) to improve the probability of obtaining the target $CD34^+$ cell dose in one collection. The use of mobilization and collection algorithms used for autologous donation has been applied to allogeneic donations to optimize collections intended for cell selection (Storch et al. 2015). For example, a peripheral blood $CD34^+$ cell count from the donor on the day prior to anticipated collection can be used to assess the level of mobilization. Poor mobilizers can be identified prior to collection and augmented with plerixafor to ensure maximal $CD34^+$ cell doses from a single collection. At centers where cell selection of National Marrow Donor Program (NMDP)-facilitated donations occurs, the option to augment mobilization with plerixafor is not available at this time. In this situation where there is a multiple day collection, one either may select the entirety of the collection or select the collection with the highest $CD34^+$ cell content and perhaps optimize the selection by adding a portion of the other product to maximally load the magnetic column. A minimum $CD34^+$ cells threshold of 2.4×10^6 cells/kg of recipient body weight is considered a *conforming product* per the package insert of the CliniMACS $CD34^+$ cell enrichment system. Therefore, depending on the degree of HLA match between the donor and recipient, a patient scheduled to receive a $CD34^+$ cell-enriched HPC product whose donor mobilizes "poorly" such that the anticipated graft will have a $CD34^+$ dose of $<2.4 \times 10^6$ $CD34^+$ cells/kg of recipient weight may need to *forego selection* in order to preserve an adequate target cell dose. Typical $CD34^+$ cell losses range from 0% to 50% in successful selection runs with 70% being an average $CD34^+$ cell recovery. Such a decision would have to be made in close collaboration with the patient's transplant physician since there are important implications for therapeutic management of the G*v*HD prophylaxis medications and subsequent risk of developing G*v*HD.

5.5 Expert Point of View

Cell selection of HPC grafts clearly has both benefits and limitations. Besides the aforementioned characteristics, cell selection has allowed the field of HCT to overcome a previously intractable hurdle, the lack of an HLA-matched donor. Historically in the absence of an HLA-matched donor or the ability to modify the HPC graft to remove alloreactive T cells via cell selection, a patient was simply not a transplant candidate, and therefore potentially lifesaving therapy was unavailable. There have however been major advances in posttransplant therapeutic strategies which allow the use of haploidentical T-cell replete HPC products with satisfactory results (Montoro et al. 2016). In fact, direct comparison of ex vivo T-cell negative selection and posttransplant cyclophosphamide (PTCy) T-cell replete haploidentical HPC graft transplants shows comparable results (Dufort et al. 2016). The use of PTCy with a T-cell replete HPC graft has several logistic and resource utilization advantages. Due to the fact that the graft, usually HPC(M) due to a lower T-cell content, would need minimal modification in the form of possible RBC and/or plasma reduction, it is substantially easier for processing facilities to accommodate at short notice. There is often clinical urgency for patients during the workup for identifying a suitable HPC donor, due to concerns for imminent relapse, and therefore it may not be clinically feasible to await an opening in the calendar to allow for cell selection. Another marked advantage is dispensing the need for complex processing and testing and technical expertise associated with cell selection, which can be financially burdensome to the medical system. Thus while it appears that new approaches which use T-cell replete grafts are in direct competition, this author would argue that they are in fact complementary strategies which expand the ability of a transplant program to serve even more patients. Depending upon the time urgency of the transplant, the resources available to the patient, the specific clinical parameters for the patient's disease (malignant vs. nonmalignant hematology indications), and either cell-selected or unmodified HPC grafts may be a more appropriate choice.

The majority of clinical experience with cell selection has centered upon CD34+ enrichment, positive selection. The intended effect, specifically marked reduction of GvHD, by passive but extensive T-cell reduction has certainly been achieved. While it appears that some previously reported limitations of cell-selected transplants like graft rejection and increased relapse risk can be compensated by the administration of "mega CD34+ cell doses" (i.e., $>10 \times 10^6$ CD34+ cells/kg of recipient body weight) and more intensive conditioning regimens with more antitumor activity, other issues remain (Aversa 2015). Of great clinical importance is the marked delay or absence of immune recovery. In order to compensate for suboptimal immune function, patients are often treated with numerous antimicrobial and antiviral agents which have the potential to contribute to myelosuppression and poor graft function. One strategy to treat patients with viral infections has been the generation and infusion of allogeneic virus-specific T cells (Papadopoulou et al. 2014); however, there are logistic and resource utilization constraints that limit their availability to a subset of large academic transplant centers. Alternatively, emerging data has shown that using a negative selection strategy to actively remove cells expressing α/β TcR can mitigate the incidence and severity of GvHD in transplant recipients. The ex vivo removal of presumptive alloreactive T cells aims to maintain the GvHD prophylaxis benefit of CD34+ cell enrichment while retaining the complement of non-HPCs which have been shown to participate in graft vs. tumor (GvT) activity, such as TcR γ/δT cells, natural killer cells, and other immune cells. Additionally, much of the preformed immunity from the donor can be granted to the recipient by transfer of the non-HPC cells which has benefit of protection from life-threatening infections (Aversa 2015).

5.6 Future Directions

The cusp of selection technology today is focused on the exploration of a transition from a CD34⁺ cell enrichment-only paradigm to one which includes negative selected grafts in place of and/or in addition to CD34⁺ cell-enriched products.

The underlying benefit of the α/β TcR negative selection is the retention of non HPC accessory cells which can facilitate G*v*T and immune recovery for which the cell doses are not clearly defined. These authors propose that in situations where α/β TcR negative cell selection fails to deliver adequate CD34⁺ cell doses, the subsequent HPC collections and selections should be performed as CD34⁺ cell enrichments. This two-pronged strategy aims to maximize the benefit of both technologies, namely, the retention of non-HPC immune cells while simultaneously removing alloreactive α/β TcR T cells and in cases where CD34⁺ cell doses are suboptimal to "back fill" with a CD34⁺ cell-enriched product. Due to the limited experience with α/β TcR negatively selected grafts, the level of G*v*HD reduction as compared to CD34⁺ cell-enriched products has not been definitely established. However, one can imagine that the presence of T cells in a graft despite being markedly reduced in α/β TcR content can lead to increased levels of G*v*HD as compared to CD34⁺ cell-enriched products; however, the benefits of superior immune recovery outweigh the G*v*HD risk. To that end, by providing the option for a CD34⁺ cell "back fill" to supplement α/β TcR negative grafts to bolster hematopoietic recovery, one can reduce the burden of T cells administered to the patient to maintain better G*v*HD prophylactic effect. One other aspect of α/β TcR *negative selection* that is not highlighted is the retention of CD34⁺ negative HPCs. Due to the fact that there is no definitive cell marker for HPCs, we are at this time unable to quantify the benefit that this may offer, but it is an intriguing question that may be answered by examining cell doses administered and resultant engraftment times for CD34⁺-enriched vs. α/β TcR-depleted grafts. Another potential application for cell selection is to modify non-G-CSF-mobilized heterogeneous mononuclear cell (MNCs) preparations such as those used for T-cell donor lymphocyte infusions (DLIs). In cases of allogeneic HCT where there is residual host chimerism, disease relapse, or uncontrolled viral infection, the use of donor-derived mononuclear cell products (donor lymphocyte infusions (DLI) or T cells) can be invoked. The major drawback from such a strategy is the infusion of potentially alloreactive T-cells into the patient which can result in G*v*HD. Cell selection of DLI using α/β TcR depletion could be used to mitigate the risk of G*v*HD while preserving the immune effects of the cell infusion. Another group recently reported (Brodszki et al. 2016) that CD45RA⁺ negative selection of DLI can be used to provide G*v*HD-mitigated cellular immunity to posttransplant patients.

Where is the field of HCT headed, and what role will cell selection play? That is an important question for which it is clear that cell selection technology has facilitated great strides in expanding the donor pool for patients and allowed for HPC transplants not requiring G*v*HD pharmacologic prophylaxis. Some of the drawbacks of cell selection such as graft rejection, increased relapse rates, and poor immune recovery have been addressed; however, the high level of resource utilization and logistic difficulties remains. Cell-selected grafts have optimal characteristics for specific patients and can result in excellent outcomes, and these authors feel that further advances in cell target selection will lead to safer more efficacious HPC transplants.

References

Avecilla ST, Marionneaux SM, Leiva TD, Tonon JA, Chan VT, Moung C et al (2016) Comparison of manual hematocrit determinations versus automated methods for hematopoietic progenitor cell apheresis products. Transfusion 56(2):528–532

Aversa F (2015) T-cell depletion: from positive selection to negative depletion in adult patients. Bone Marrow Transplant 50(Suppl 2):S11–S13

Brodszki N, Turkiewicz D, Toporski J, Truedsson L, Dykes J (2016) Novel treatment of severe combined immunodeficiency utilizing ex-vivo T-cell depleted haploidentical hematopoietic stem cell transplantation and CD45RA+ depleted donor lymphocyte infusions. Orphanet J Rare Dis 11:5

Daniele N, Scerpa MC, Caniglia M, Bernardo ME, Rossi C, Ciammetti C et al (2012) Transplantation in the onco-hematology field: focus on the manipulation of alphabeta and gammadelta T cells. Pathol Res Pract 208(2):67–73

Doherty PC (1992) The function of gamma delta T cells. Br J Haematol 81(3):321–324

Drobyski WR, Majewski D, Hanson G (1999) Graft-facilitating doses of ex vivo activated gammadelta T cells do not cause lethal murine graft-vs.-host disease. Biol Blood Marrow Transplant 5(4):222–230

Dufort G, Castillo L, Pisano S, Castiglioni M, Carolina P, Andrea I et al (2016) Haploidentical hematopoietic stem cell transplantation in children with high-risk hematologic malignancies: outcomes with two different strategies for GvHD prevention. Ex vivo T-cell depletion and post-transplant cyclophosphamide: 10 years of experience at a single center. Bone Marrow Transplant 51(10):1354–1360

FDA (2014) Minimal manipulation of human cells, tissues, and cellular and tissue-based products: draft guidance. FDA [cited 27 Aug 2016]. http://www.fda.gov/BiologicsBloodVaccines/GuidanceComplianceRegulatoryInformation/Guidances/CellularandGeneTherapy/ucm427692.htm

Gattillo S, Marktel S, Rizzo L, Malato S, Malabarba L, Coppola M et al (2015) Plerixafor on demand in ten healthy family donors as a rescue strategy to achieve an adequate graft for stem cell transplantation. Transfusion 55(8):1993–2000

Geyer MB, Ricci AM, Jacobson JS, Majzner R, Duffy D, Van de Ven C et al (2012) T cell depletion utilizing CD34(+) stem cell selection and CD3(+) addback from unrelated adult donors in paediatric allogeneic stem cell transplantation recipients. Br J Haematol 157(2):205–219

Hauge AW, Haastrup EK, Sengelov H, Minulescu L, Dickmeiss E, Fischer-Nielsen A (2014) Addition of plerixafor for CD34+ cell mobilization in six healthy stem cell donors ensured satisfactory grafts for transplantation. Transfusion 54(4):1055–1058

Keever-Taylor CA, Devine SM, Soiffer RJ, Mendizabal A, Carter S, Pasquini MC et al (2012) Characteristics of CliniMACS(R) system CD34-enriched T cell-depleted grafts in a multicenter trial for acute myeloid leukemia-blood and marrow transplant clinical trials network (BMT CTN) protocol 0303. Biol Blood Marrow Transplant 18(5):690–697

Lamb LS Jr, Henslee-Downey PJ, Parrish RS, Godder K, Thompson J, Lee C et al (1996) Increased frequency of TCR gamma delta + T cells in disease-free survivors following T cell-depleted, partially mismatched, related donor bone marrow transplantation for leukemia. J Hematother 5(5):503–509

Montoro J, Sanz J, Sanz GF, Sanz MA (2016) Advances in haploidentical stem cell transplantation for hematologic malignancies. Leuk Lymphoma 57(8):1766–1775

Nadeau M, George L, Yeager AM, Anwer F, McBride A (2015) Plerixafor as a salvage mobilization strategy for haploidentical peripheral blood allogeneic stem cell transplantation. Clin Case Rep 3(9):728–730

Papadopoulou A, Gerdemann U, Katari UL, Tzannou I, Liu H, Martinez C et al (2014) Activity of broad-spectrum T cells as treatment for AdV, EBV, CMV, BKV, and HHV6 infections after HSCT. Sci Transl Med 6(242):242ra83

Storch E, Mark T, Avecilla S, Pagan C, Rhodes J, Shore T et al (2015) A novel hematopoietic progenitor cell mobilization and collection algorithm based on preemptive CD34 enumeration. Transfusion 55(8):2010–2016

Teschner D, Distler E, Wehler D, Frey M, Marandiuc D, Langeveld K et al (2014) Depletion of naive T cells using clinical grade magnetic CD45RA beads: a new approach for GVHD prophylaxis. Bone Marrow Transplant 49(1):138–144

Theilgaard-Monch K, Raaschou-Jensen K, Schjodt K, Heilmann C, Vindelov L, Jacobsen N et al (2003) Pluripotent and myeloid-committed CD34+ subsets in hematopoietic stem cell allografts. Bone Marrow Transplant 32(12):1125–1133

Cryopreservation Techniques and Freezing Solutions

6

Rona Singer Weinberg

6.1 Introduction

Hematopoietic progenitor cell (HPC) products remain viable and capable of engraftment in a transplant recipient when stored in the "liquid state" at either refrigerated or room temperatures for approximately 72 h following collection. Cryopreservation enables long-term storage of HPC products and is used extensively for autologous products collected prior to high-dose chemotherapy (HDT) that are intended for use after treatment to rescue hematopoiesis. Allogeneic products may also be cryopreserved if treatment is delayed due to the donor's or recipient's medical condition, the donor's cells are collected prior to their anticipated use because of donor availability, or more donor cells are obtained than needed and remaining cells are stored for future use. Similarly, allogeneic cord blood products are cryopreserved, prospectively banked, and made available through donor registries. In order for cryopreservation to be an effective tool, when thawed and infused, HPC must be able to regain their ability to proliferate, engraft, and provide the same functional capability as prior to cryopreservation. Pre-cryopreservation storage conditions and manipulation procedures, cryoprotectant formulation, freezing rate, long-term storage temperatures, length of time in storage, and thawing conditions all have the potential to affect the quality and engraftment of thawed HPC products.

R.S. Weinberg, Ph.D.
Cellular Therapy Laboratory, New York Blood Center, New York, NY, USA
e-mail: rweinberg@nybloodcenter.org

J. Schwartz, B.H. Shaz (eds.), *Best Practices in Processing and Storage for Hematopoietic Cell Transplantation*, Advances and Controversies in Hematopoietic Transplantation and Cell Therapy,
https://doi.org/10.1007/978-3-319-58949-7_6

6.2 Pre-cryopreservation Transport, Storage, and Processing Considerations

The temperature(s) at which HPC products are stored and transported prior to processing, manufacturing, and cryopreservation can influence the viability, sterility, potency, efficacy, and overall quality of the products. However, "standard" temperatures have not been established. Storage and transport temperature(s) vary by collection and manufacturing facility, and some facilities even use different temperatures for products collected from different sources (e.g., apheresis, marrow, and cord blood) (Antonenas et al. 2006; Hahn et al. 2014; Lazarus et al. 2009; Fry et al. 2013; Kao et al. 2011). These temperatures range from refrigeration (2–10 °C) to ambient or room temperatures (up to 20 °C). Even the National Marrow Donor Program (NMDP, Be the Match®), which transports more than 6000 HPC products annually from collection centers to transplant centers throughout the world, *does not* have a standard transport temperature but rather leaves storage and transport conditions to the discretion of the transplant center.

Minimal manipulations of HPC products, such as plasma and red blood cell reduction, are often performed prior to cryopreservation. Plasma reduction rarely results in significant cell loss; however, red blood cell reduction may result in loss of as many as 30% of total nucleated cells (TNCs). Removal of donor red blood cells and/or plasma effectively reduces the risks of hemolysis associated with donor and recipient ABO/Rh incompatibility. The volume of cryoprotectant used is proportional to the volume of the product. Removing red blood cells and/or plasma reduces the volume of the product and also serves to reduce the volume of cryoprotectant in the cryopreserved product, thus reducing the risks of infusion adverse reactions attributable to the concentration of cryoprotectant administered to the patient. From a practical standpoint, the reduced total volume also conserves reagents, cryopreservation bags, and valuable freezer storage space. More than minimal manipulation such as $CD34^+$ cell enrichment and $CD3^+$ cell reduction with monoclonal antibodies and ex vivo expansion cultures may make HPC more susceptible to damage during cryopreservation, and thawing and cryopreservation protocols may or may not need to be modified to improve recovery of these much needed cells (Gorin 1986; Reich-Slotky et al. 2016) (Table 6.1).

6.3 Cellular Composition and Concentration

HPC, Marrow and *HPC, Apheresis* differs significantly in cell content and volume. HPC, Marrow contains a large proportion of mature granulocytes and red blood cells which lyse when cryopreserved and thawed. The lysed cells and the toxic materials released can cause serious infusion complications including renal failure and, in rare instances, death (Rowley 1992). Historically, *HPC, Marrow* products were processed and cryopreserved prior to the advent of *HPC, Apheresis* collections. Based on experience with *HPC, Marrow*, cell concentrations up to 1×10^8 nucleated cells (NCs)/mL in a cryoprotectant containing 10% dimethylsulfoxide (DMSO, volume/volume) were suggested for cryopreserved products (Rowley 1992; Cabezudo et al. 2000;

Table 6.1 Pre-cryopreservation storage and processing considerations

Condition	Risks
Liquid storage temperature	Refrigeration temperatures may reduce viability Room temperature may increase the risk of microbial contamination
Plasma reduction	Reduces hemolysis risk due to minor ABO/Rh incompatibility Reduces concentration of DMSO required, thereby reducing risks of infusion adverse reactions Minimal cell loss
RBC reduction	Reduces red cell lysis during thawing, thereby reducing infusion adverse events Reduces hemolysis risk due to donor and recipient major ABO/Rh incompatibility Cell loss may be significant (≥30% total nucleated cells)
Cell concentration	*HPC, Marrow* has lower cell counts than HPC, Apheresis Large dilutions can result in large volumes of DMSO which may cause adverse reactions when infused
Cell enrichment (or reduction), e.g., CD34$^+$ cell enrichment (or CD3$^+$ cell reduction	Reduced cell viability and recovery Cells may be more sensitive to DMSO
Cell types to be recovered	HPC may be more resistant to cryopreservation than lymphocytes
Ex vivo culture/expansion	Increased apoptosis Culture media may improve viability due to amino acids, protein, and antioxidants

Rowley et al. 1994). However, *HPC, Apheresis* can contain as many as fivefold more cells making dilution to similar cell concentrations impractical since these dilutions would result in very large volumes that are difficult to store and infuse and contain large volumes of DMSO which can be toxic (Gorin 1986). Recovery of nucleated and CD34$^+$ cells, clonogenic assays, and engraftment have been used to compare *HPC, Apheresis* products cryopreserved at low and high cell concentrations (Cabezudo et al. 2000; Rowley et al. 1994; Lecchi et al. 2016; Martin-Henao et al. 2005). In these studies, *HPC, Apheresis* was cryopreserved at concentrations up to approximately fourfold the recommended *HPC, Marrow* concentrations. In all instances, the concentration of cells at the time of cryopreservation did not significantly affect the post-thaw recovery of HPC or the time to engraftment of these cells.

6.4 Cryoprotectants

Cryoprotectants are added to HPC products prior to cryopreservation in order to limit cell lysis during the cooling/freezing process (Gorin 1986). DMSO, a small molecule that diffuses into cells, is the most commonly used cryoprotectant.

Intracellular DMSO changes the osmotic balance of cells and interferes with ice crystal formation, thereby reducing cell lysis and preserving cell viability (Rowley 1992; Lecchi et al. 2016; Karow and Webb 1965). Because cryopreservation in DMSO decreased the proliferative potential of bone marrow progenitor cell colonies in some studies, it has been assumed that DMSO is toxic to HPC and that exposure to DMSO in the non-cryopreserved state (Douay et al. 1982) and post-thaw (Rowley 1992) should be limited. However, colony-forming progenitor cells were resistant to toxic effects of up to 20% DMSO for up to 1 h (Rowley and Anderson 1993) and 8–10% DMSO for at least 2 h (Branch et al. 1994). DMSO is generally diluted in an isotonic solution containing a source of protein such as human serum albumin or autologous plasma (Rowley 1992; Smagur et al. 2015). Concentrations ranging from 3.5% to 10% DMSO maintain HPC viability and have been reported to have similar engraftment outcomes when products are thawed and infused (Rowley 1992; Smagur et al. 2015; Lovelock and Bishop 1959; Veeraputhiran et al. 2010; Fry et al. 2015; Stiff et al. 1987).

DMSO does not protect red blood cells and granulocytes in HPC products from lysis during freezing and thawing. Lysis of these cells, and the toxic materials that they release (hemoglobin and nucleoprotein and lysosomal enzymes, respectively), has been implicated in infusion adverse reactions. Hydroxyethyl starch (HES) is a high-molecular-weight extracellular cryoprotectant that reduces post-thaw granulocyte lysis and clumping (Stiff et al. 1987). Addition of 6% HES to DMSO enables cryopreservation at a lower DMSO concentration (5%) and lowers granulocyte lysis, both of which reduce the occurrence of infusion adverse reactions without compromising viability and engraftment of HPC (Stiff et al. 1987). Dextran 40, another high-molecular-weight extracellular cryoprotectant, has been used extensively for cryopreservation of HPC, Cord Blood. Addition of dextran 40 to the cryoprotectant reduces DMSO toxicity during the cooling process (Rubinstein et al. 1995).

Because DMSO can be toxic to cells and may cause infusion-related adverse events, a non-DMSO-containing cryoprotectant may be advantageous. HPC cryopreserved in DMSO and the low-molecular-weight carbohydrate Pentaisomaltose (PIM) were compared (Svalgaard et al. 2016). Post-thaw, cells were analyzed for $CD34^+$ cell recovery and viability, and $CD34^+$ cell subsets by flow cytometry; and in vitro colony assays were also performed. All analyses indicated that PIM was comparable to DMSO as a cryoprotectant and therefore may have the potential to be used as a less toxic cryoprotectant. Preclinical, in vivo animal studies will be needed to confirm these findings prior to clinical studies.

Although cryopreserved HPC products have been used clinically for decades, successful cryopreservation and subsequent clinical use of other cellular therapy products have been more challenging and may require modification of procedures and cryopreservative formulations. Aliquots of allogeneic *HPC, Apheresis* products may be cryopreserved as a source of donor lymphocytes for infusion if indicated to treat relapse or speed immune recovery posttransplant making stability and recovery of white blood cells critical (Stroncek et al. 2011). The post-thaw recovery and viability of HPC and lymphocytes cryopreserved under standard conditions were compared (Fisher et al. 2014; Berens et al. 2016). In one study (Fisher et al. 2014), $CD34^+$ cell recovery from related and unrelated donors was similar; however, $CD3^+$ cell recovery was lower in products from unrelated donors. Since all unrelated donors had undergone mobilization with G-CSF while many related donors had not, products from mobilized related and unrelated donors were also compared. Recovery of $CD3^+$ cells was found to be similar in both groups, indicating that donor mobilization with G-CSF may have a negative effect on recovery of $CD3^+$ cells post-cryopreservation. Another study (Berens et al. 2016) demonstrated that recovery of cryopreserved $CD3^+$ cells and $CD4^+$ and $CD8^+$ subsets was decreased compared to recovery of $CD34^+$ cells. In this study, there was no correlation between lymphocyte recovery and donor mobilization with G-CSF, and the investigators concluded that resistance to freezing and thawing is cell specific and independent of other factors. Ex vivo expanded HPC, Cord Blood survives poorly when cryopreserved using standard procedures. Addition of serum-free culture medium containing carbohydrates and antioxidants improved the recovery of viable HPC as evidenced by decreased apoptosis, increased numbers of in vitro progenitor cell assays, and engraftment in primary and secondary immunodeficient NSG mice (Duchez et al. 2016).

6.5 Cooling Process: Controlled Versus Passive Rate Freezing

HPC must be cooled slowly in order to preserve post-thaw viability and function. Many transplant centers use controlled rate freezers to cryopreserve these products (Rowley 1992). The programmed freeze cycle consists of *three phases*. The first is the equilibrium phase during which the product is cooled to the same temperature as the freezing chamber. This ensures that the product's temperature can be monitored accurately throughout the process to provide freezing curve uniformity for all products. A constant cooling rate is achieved during the second phase. The optimal cooling rate for HPC products is 1–2 °C/min. Extracellular ice formation which is an exothermic reaction occurs during this phase, and the program must compensate for the heat that is released. This is usually accomplished by an "ice seeding" procedure whereby the product is cooled very quickly and then warmed slightly before continuing the constant cooling rate. Extracellular ice formation decreases the available water in the extracellular space, thereby increasing the extracellular concentration and efflux of water from the cells can occur. Decreasing the temperature at which extracellular ice formation occurs protects cellular viability. In the final phase, cooling continues at a constant rate until the desired temperature is achieved (Hubel 2009).

Controlled rate freezing (CRF) requires costly equipment and cooling program development. Once the cooling cycle is started, controlled rate freezers cannot be opened to add additional products. As a result, processing labs must either have multiple freezers or coordinate processing of multiple products so that all can be placed in the freezer at the same time assuring minimal exposure time (usually <15 min) to DMSO prior to cooling process. As a less expensive, rapid, easy, and very reproducible alternative, "dump" or "passive" freezing has been developed and is used extensively (Stiff et al. 1987; Halle et al. 2001; Detry et al. 2014). Products in metal freezing cassettes are placed horizontally on shelves in a −80 °C mechanical freezer. The freezing rate can be monitored easily by placing the probe of an electronic temperature monitor inside the cassette, against the cryopreservation bag. The metal cassette can be wrapped in disposable absorbent pads or Styrofoam insulation to adjust the cooling rate to the desired 1–2 °C/min. Cell viability, recovery, and engraftment are comparable to CRF.

6.6 Long-Term Storage Temperatures and Hematopoietic Progenitor Cell Stability

Cryopreserved HPC products may remain in storage for prolonged periods of time. In order to provide adequate HPC for successful hematopoietic cell transplantation, the stability and potency of these products must be maintained during storage. Most clinical facilities store HPC products in the liquid or vapor phases of liquid nitrogen (−195 °C or −150 to −125 °C, respectively), and successful storage at −80 °C in mechanical freezers has also been reported (Halle et al. 2001; Detry et al. 2014). It has not been determined if viability and engraftment potential is increased by storage in the liquid phase of nitrogen versus the vapor phase. Accreditation standards organizations such as NetCord-FACT/JACIE (Foundation for the Accreditation of Cellular Therapy and International NetCord Foundation 2016) require *HPC, Cord Blood* to be stored at temperatures ≤−150 °C because of the assumption that a lower temperature will better maintain the stability and viability of the products over extended periods of storage experienced by public cord blood banks. Because temperature gradients can occur in liquid nitrogen vapor resulting in temperatures ≥−150 °C toward the top of vessel, many cord blood banks have chosen to store products in the liquid phase. A major disadvantage to storage in the liquid phase is the potential transmission of infectious disease and microbial contamination between products if cryopreservation bags in which products are stored do not remain intact (Tedder et al. 1995; Fountain et al. 1997). Storage in liquid nitrogen vapor phase eliminates this risk. Storage at −80 °C in mechanical freezers may not be sufficient for storage longer than approximately 2 years and may result in loss of products due to mechanical failure (Halle et al. 2001; Detry et al. 2014). Assays used to evaluate post-thaw product functionality include comparison of pre-cryopreservation and post-thaw viable total nucleated and $CD34^+$ cells by flow cytometry, in vitro progenitor cell colony growth and replating efficiencies, engraftment in animal models such as immunodeficient mice, and derivation of induced pluripotent stem cells that can differentiate into all three germ layers (Broxmeyer et al. 2003, 2011; Vosganian et al. 2012; Winter et al. 2014). Ultimately, engraftment in human subjects is the most important indicator of product stability. Cryopreserved *HPC, Apheresis* and *HPC, Cord Blood* have been evaluated and remain viable and function for at least 15 and 23.5 years, respectively (Broxmeyer et al. 2003, 2011; Vosganian et al. 2012; Winter et al. 2014).

6.7 Potential Infusion-Related Adverse Events from Thawed Products

Cryopreserved products are generally thawed quickly, often at the patient's bedside, and infused immediately to limit exposure of HPC to DMSO at warm temperatures. Procedures for thawing, washing, and preparing products for infusion are discussed in detail in Chaps. 7 and 11 of this book.

Adverse events can occur during infusion of thawed products. These reactions are generally mild and have been attributed to reactions to DMSO (Zambelli et al. 1998; Davis et al. 1990; Stroncek et al. 1991; Donmez et al. 2007), lysis of red blood cells and the resultant release of hemoglobin (Smith et al. 1987), and release of nucleoprotein and lysosomal enzymes by lysis of granulocytes (Davis et al. 1990) during the freezing and thawing process. Reported mild to moderate infusion-related adverse events include nausea and vomiting, headache, hypotension, bradycardia, tachycardia, chest tightness, fever and chills, and abdominal cramps. Less frequently, renal failure and severe cardiac and neurologic symptoms have been reported. Severe cardiac side effects require the infusion to be stopped and have been attributed to high DMSO and cell concentrations in the product (Donmez et al. 2007). In order to limit DMSO-related toxicity, infusion of DMSO should be limited to <1 g DMSO/kg of recipient body weight (Rowley et al. 1994).

6.8 Expert Point of View

HPC products have been cryopreserved by transplant centers for many years. Despite the universality of cryopreservation, there is no standard or even consensus with regard to the final cell or DMSO concentrations or other additives used (Table 6.2). However, it is generally agreed that addition of DMSO together with a slow cooling/freezing rate limits intracellular ice crystal formation and cell lysis, thereby preserving cell viability. Similarly, successful long-term storage has been reported at temperatures ranging from −196 to −80 °C. Rapid bedside thawing and immediate infusion to limit post-thaw exposure of cells to DMSO have been adopted by most centers. Fortunately, cryopreserved HPC are very robust and resilient and have been shown to be stable regardless of the technical variations reported and can be stored and remain viable, capable of engraftment, and available for patients for at least 20 years.

Table 6.2 Variable cryopreservation conditions

Cryoprotectants	3.5–10% DMSO in isotonic solution (saline, normosol, or culture media); ±serum (autologous or human serum albumin); ±hespan; ±dextran 40.
Cooling	Controlled rate versus passive; 1–2 °C/min
Temperature	*Liquid* phase of nitrogen (−195 °C), *vapor* phase of nitrogen (≤−150 °C), mechanical freezers (−80 °C)
Stability	Up to 23.5 years for CBU and 15 years for HPC, Apheresis

6.9 Future Directions

Manufacture of gene and immunotherapy products involves more than minimal manipulation and long-term ex vivo cultures. These processes may render cells more fragile and sensitive to current cryopreservation procedures. In order to make these products available to most patients, methods will have to be modified to protect the viability and functionality of complex cellular therapy products.

References

Antonenas V, Garvin F, Webb M, Sartor M, Bradstock KF, Gottlieb D (2006) Fresh PBSC harvests, but not BM, show temperature-related loss of CD 34 viability during storage and transport. Cytotherapy 8:158–165

Berens C, Heine A, Muller J, Held SAE, Mayer K, Brossart P, Oldenburg J, Potzch B, Wolf D, Ruhl H (2016) Variable resistance to freezing and thawing of CD34-postivie stem cells and lymphocyte subpopulations in leukapheresis products. Cytotherapy 18:1325–1331

Branch DR, Calderwood S, Cecutti MA, Herst R, Solh H (1994) Hematopoietic progenitor cells are resistant to dimethyl sulfoxide toxicity. Transfusion 34:887–890

Broxmeyer HE, Srour EF, Hangoc G, Cooper S, Anderson SA, Bodine DM (2003) High-efficiency recovery of functional hematopoietic progenitor and stem cells from human cord blood cryopreserved for 15 years. Proc Natl Acad Sci U S A 100:645–650

Broxmeyer HE, Lee M-R, Hangoc G, Cooper S, Prasain N, Kim Y-J, Mallet C, Ye Z, Witting S, Cornetta K, Cheng L, Yoder MC (2011) Hematopoietic stem/progenitor cells, generation of induced pluripotent stem cells and isolation of endothelial progenitors from 21- to 23.5-year cryopreserved cord blood. Blood 117:4774–4777

Cabezudo E, Dalmases C, Ruiz M, Sanchez JA, Torrico C, Sola C et al (2000) Leukapheresis components may be cryopreserved at high cell concentrations without additional loss of HPC function. Transfusion 40:1223–1227

Davis JM, Rowley SD, Braine HG, Piantadosi S, Santos GW (1990) Clinical toxicity of cryopreserved bone marrow graft infusion. Blood 75:781–786

Detry G, Calvet L, Straetmans N, Cabrespine A, Ravoet C, Bay JO, Petre H, Paillard C, Husson B, Merlin E, Boon-Falleur L, Tournilhac O, Delannoy A, Halle P (2014) Impact of uncontrolled freezing and long-term storage of peripheral blood stem cells at −80 °C on haematopoietic recovery after autologous transplantation. Report from two centres. Bone Marrow Transplant 49:780–785

Donmez A, Tombuloglu M, Gungor A, Soyer N, Saydam G, Cagirgan S (2007) Clinical side effects during peripheral blood progenitor cell infusion. Transfus Apher Sci 36:95–101

Douay L, Gorin NC, David R et al (1982) Study of granulocyte-macrophage progenitor (CFUc) preservation after slow freezing of bone marrow in the gas phase of liquid nitrogen. Exp Hematol 10:360–366

Duchez P, Rodriguez L, Chevaleyre J, DeLaGrange PB, Ivanovic Z (2016) Clinical-scale validation of a new efficient procedure for cryopreservation of ex vivo expanded cord blood hematopoietic stem and progenitor cells. Cytotherapy 18:1543–1547

Fisher V, Khuu H, David-OCampo V, Byrne K Pavletic S, Bishop M, Fowler DH, Barrett AJ, Stroncek DF (2014) Analysis of the recovery of cryopreserved and thawed CD34+ and CD3+cells collected for hematopoietic transplantation. Transfusion 54:1088–1092

Foundation for the Accreditation of Cellular Therapy and International NetCord Foundation (2016) NetCord-FACT international cord blood standards accreditation manual, 6th edn. Foundation for the Accreditation of Cellular Therapy and International NetCord Foundation, Nebraska, p 157

Fountain D, Ralston M, Higgins N, Gorlin JB, Uhl L, Wheeler C et al (1997) Liquid nitrogen freezers: a potential source of microbial contamination of hematopoietic stem cell components. Transfusion 37:585–591

Fry LJ, Giner SQ, Gomez SG, Green M, Anderson F, Horder J, McArdle S, Rees R, Madrigal JA (2013) Avoiding room temperature storage and delayed cryopreservation provide better post-thaw potency in hematopoietic progenitor cell grafts. Transfusion 53:1834–1842

Fry LJ, Querol S, Gomez SG, McArdle S, Rees R, Madrigal JA (2015) Assessing the toxic effects of DMSO on cord blood to determine exposure time limits and the optimum concentration for cryopreservation. Vox Sang 109:181–190

Gorin NC (1986) Collection, manipulation and freezing of haemopoietic stem cells. Clin Haematol 15:19–48

Hahn S, Sireis W, Hourfar K, Karpova D, Dauber K, Kempf VAJ, Selfried E, Schmidt M, Bonig H (2014) Effects of storage temperature on hematopoietic stability and microbial safety of BM aspirates. Bone Marrow Transplant 49:338–348

Halle P, Tournihac O, Knopinsk-Posluszny W, Kanold J, Gembara P, Boiret N, Rapatel C, Berger M, Travade P, Angielski S, Bonhomme J, Demeocq F (2001) Uncontrolled-rate freezing and storage at −80°C, with only 3.5 percent DMSO in cryoprotective solution for 109 autologous peripheral blood progenitor cell transplantations. Transfusion 41:667–672

Hubel A (2009) Cryopreservation of cellular therapy products. In: Areman EM, Loper K (eds) Cellular therapy: principles, methods, and regulations. Maryland, AABB, pp p342–p357

Kao GS, Kim HT, Daley H, Ritz J, Burger SR, Kelly L, Vierra-Green C, Flesch S, Spellman S, Miller J, Confer D (2011) Validation of short-term handling and storage conditions for marrow and peripheral blood stem cell products. Transfusion 51:137–147

Karow AM Jr, Webb WR (1965) Tissue freezing a theory for injury and survival. Cryobiology 2:99–108

Lazarus HM, Kan F, Tarima S, Champlin RE, Confer DL, Frey N, Gee AP, Wagner JE, Horowitz MM, Eapen M (2009) Rapid transport and infusion of hematopoietic cells is associated with improved outcome after myeloablative therapy and unrelated donor transplant. Biol Blood Marrow Transplant 15:589–596

Lecchi L, Giovanelli S, Gagliardi B, Pezzali I, Ratti I, Marconi M (2016) An update on methods for cryopreservation and thawing of hemopoietic stem cells. Transfus Apher Sci 54:324–336

Lovelock JE, Bishop MWH (1959) Prevention of freezing damage to living cells by dimethyl sulfoxide. Nature 183:1394–1395

Martin-Henao GA, Torrico C, Azueta C, Amill B, Querol S, Garcia J (2005) Cryopreservation of hematopoietic progenitor cells from apheresis at high cell concentrations does not impair the hematopoietic recovery after transplantation. Transfusion 45:1917–1924

Reich-Slotky R, Bachegowda LS, Ancharski M, Gergis U, van Besien K, Cushing MM (2016) Engraftment for CD34 selected stem cell products is not compromised by cryopreservation. Transfusion 56:893–898

Rowley SD (1992) Hematopoietic stem cell cryopreservation: a review of current techniques. J Hematother 1:233–250

Rowley SD, Anderson GL (1993) Effect of DMSO exposure without cryopreservation on hematopoietic progenitor cells. Bone Marrow Transplant 11:389–393

Rowley SD, Bensinger WI, Gooley TA, Buckner CD (1994) Effect of cell concentration on bone marrow and peripheral blood stem cell cryopreservation. Blood 83:2731–2736

Rubinstein P, Dobrila L, Rosenfield RE, Adamson JW, Migliaccio G, Migliaccio AR, Taylor PE, Stevens CE (1995) Processing and cryopreservation of placental/umbilical cord blood for unrelated bone marrow reconstitution. Proc Natl Acad Sci U S A 92:10119–10122

Smagur A, Mitrus I, Ciomber A, Panczyniak K, Fidyk W, Sadus-Wojciechowska M, Holowiecki J, Giebel S (2015) Comparison of cryoprotective solutions based on human albumin vs. autologous plasma: its effect on cell recovery, clonogenic potential of peripheral blood hematopoietic progenitor cells and engraftment after autologous transplantation. Vox Sang 108: 417–424

Smith DM, Weisenburger DD, Bierman P, Kessinger A, Vaughan WP, Armitage JO (1987) Acute renal failure associated with autologous bone marrow transplantation. Bone Marrow Transplant 2:195

Stiff PJ, Koester AR, Weidner MK, Dvorak K, Fisher RI (1987) Autologous bone marrow transplantation using unfractionated cells cryopreserved in dimethylsulfoxide and hydroxyethyl starch without controlled-rate freezing. Blood 70:974–978

Stroncek DF, Fautsch SK, Lasky LC, Hurd DD, Ramsay NKC, McCullough J (1991) Adverse reactions in patients transfused with cryopreserved marrow. Transfusion 31:521–526

Stroncek DE, Xing L, Chau Q, Zia N, McKelvy A, Pracht L, Sabatino M, Jin P (2011) Stability of cryopreserved white blood cells (WBCs) prepared for donor WBC infusions. Tranfusion 51:2647–2655

Svalgaard JD, Haastrup EK, Reckzeh K, Holst B, Glovinski PV, Gorlov JS, Hansen MB, Moench KT, Clausen C, Fischer-Nielsen A (2016) Low-molecular-weight carbohydrate Pentaisomaltose may replace dimethyl sulfoxide as a safer cryoprotectant for cryopreservation of peripheral blood stem cells. Transfusion 56:1088–1095

Tedder RS, FFuckerman MA, Goldstone AH, Hawkins AE, Fielding A, Briggs EM et al (1995) Hepatitis B transmission from contaminated cryopreservation tank. Lancet 346:137–140

Veeraputhiran M, Theus JW, Pesek G, Barlogie B, Cottler-Fox M (2010) Viability and engraftment of hematopoietic progenitor cells after long-term cryopreservation: effect of diagnosis and percentage dimethyl sulfoxide concentration. Cytotherapy 12:764–766

Vosganian GS, Waalen J, Kim K, Jhatakia S, Scram E, Lee T, Riddell D, Mason JR (2012) Effects of long-term cryopreservation on peripheral blood progenitor cells. Cytotherapy 14:1228–1234

Winter JM, Jacobson P, Bullough B, Christensen AP, Boyer M, Reems J-A (2014) Long-erm effects of cryopreservation on clinically prepared hematopoietic progenitor cell products. Cytotherapy 16:965–975

Zambelli A, Poggi G, Da Prada G, Pedrazzoli P, Cuomo A, Miotti D, Perotti C, Preti P, Robustelli della Cuna G (1998) Clinical toxicity of cryopreserved circulating progenitor cells infusion. Anticancer Res 18:4705–4708

Peripheral Blood Hematopoietic Progenitor Cell Graft Thawing

7

Ronit Reich-Slotky

7.1 Introduction

The use of peripheral blood (PB) as the cell source for hematopoietic cell transplant (HCT) has been steadily replacing the use of bone marrow (BM). Mobilized PB is the major source of HPC for autologous hematopoietic cell transplants (auto-HCT) and is currently being used for more than 75% of adult related and unrelated allogeneic hematopoietic cell transplants (allo-HCT) (Pasquini and Zhu 2015). The number of autologous and allogeneic transplants in the USA and worldwide is constantly increasing, and the use of PB HPCs in the allogeneic transplant setting is increasing as well, despite its higher risk of graft-versus-host disease (G*v*HD) compared to BM grafts. The composition of PB products is different from the traditional BM. They typically contain two- to fivefold more $CD34^+$ progenitor cells and tenfold more T-cells. The collection by apheresis results in a relatively smaller volume with significantly lower red blood cell (RBC) volume (Snyder and Haley 2004; Kao 2009). Due to the high $CD34^+$ content, PB products provide much faster hematological reconstitution than BM or Cord Blood (CB). Development of new pharmacologic mobilization agents allowed graft collection from patients previously unable to mobilize enough HPC, thereby increasing the potential number of total collections and transplants (Brave et al. 2010; Keating 2011).

R. Reich-Slotky, Ph.D., M.Sc.
Department of Transfusion Medicine and Cellular Therapy, New York Presbyterian Hospital - Weill Cornell Medical Center, New York, NY, USA
e-mail: Ros9085@nyp.org

J. Schwartz, B.H. Shaz (eds.), *Best Practices in Processing and Storage for Hematopoietic Cell Transplantation*, Advances and Controversies in Hematopoietic Transplantation and Cell Therapy,
https://doi.org/10.1007/978-3-319-58949-7_7

7.2 Cryopreservation of Peripheral Blood Graft

The stability of fresh cellular products is time sensitive, and, if done properly, cryopreservation allows long-term storage of viable and potent HPCs. For autologous donors, cryopreservation is essential, allowing advanced collection of cells for later auto-HCT. This also allows collecting and storing enough cells for possible multiple future transplants, which is a common practice for multiple myeloma (MM) patients. The use of cryopreservation of HPC for allo-HCT is not as common. PB HPCs are collected from related or unrelated donors and are typically infused fresh, within <72 h of apheresis collection. The National Marrow Donor Program (NMDP) requires products from non-related donors to be used fresh, and any cryopreservation requires additional approval. However, cryopreservation can be a powerful tool for allogeneic products as well. Often the donor availability is limited due to the need to travel or other restrictions, or the transplant has to be delayed after the donor has already been mobilized for HPC. Additionally, any product leftovers can be stored for possible future use, thus eliminating the need to re-collect the donor, i.e., donor T lymphocytes.

To allow long-term storage, PB procured HPC products are usually cooled slowly at a controlled rate (see Chap. 6) and stored below −150 °C in a *vapor phase* liquid nitrogen (LN2) freezer. The most commonly used cryoprotectant is dimethyl sulfoxide (DMSO), but other molecules, such as hydroxyethyl starch (HES), are used in combination with DMSO. HES is a high-molecular-weight polymer that does not penetrate cells and is used clinically as plasma expander in hypotensive patients (Vercueil et al. 2005). It can stabilize RBC and reduce the sudden changes in osmolality that occur when thawing cryopreserved cells. Adverse events associated with HES are rare, and it was recently shown not to have an association with adverse events which were previously described (Bothner et al. 1998; Wagner et al. 2002; Pagano et al. 2016). A typical cryopreservation media comprises of an isotonic solution containing protein source, such as donor plasma or commercially available human serum albumin (HSA), and 5–10% DMSO. Prolonged storage duration was not shown to affect HPC potency, and many studies have shown that cryopreserved HPC can retain engraftment potential for more than a decade (Spurr et al. 2002; Donnenberg et al. 2002; Broxmeyer et al. 2003; Foïs et al. 2007).

7.3 DMSO Toxicity and Cryopreservation-Related Infusion Adverse Events

Cryopreservation can induce cell damage due to ice formation and dehydration (Mazur et al. 1972). Lovelock and Bishop described the properties and use of DMSO for cryopreservation of living cells (Lovelock and Bishop 1959). DMSO is a rapid penetrating molecule that increases the tolerance of cells to the osmotic stress induced by cryopreservation. It was originally used as an anti-inflammatory reagent but was later found to cause an array of side effects when administered to patients (Yellowlees et al. 1980; Runckel and Swanson 1980; Samoszuk et al. 1983). DMSO toxicity in HPC product infusion was shown to affect multiple organs including respiratory, cardiovascular, gastrointestinal, hepatic, and renal systems. Side effects related to infusion of thawed products are usually mild or moderate, most commonly nausea, vomiting, and hypertension. Other side effects such as abdominal cramps, chills, flushing, headaches, and diarrhea have been reported as well (Zambelli et al. 1998; Alessandrino et al. 1999; Sauer-Heilborn et al. 2004; Davis et al. 1990). Severe side effects are rare, but cardiovascular, neurological, and respiratory side effects have been reported, with some of them being severe or fatal (Windrum et al. 2005; Benekli et al. 2000; Zenhäusern et al. 2000; Rapoport et al. 1991; Hoyt et al. 2000; Dhodapkar et al. 1994; Smith et al. 1987). The rate of side effects was shown to correlate with increase in DMSO volume (Davis et al. 1990). Beside DMSO toxicity, thawed products contain cell debris, toxin, and free hemoglobin, and all of these substances can induce side effects when administered to patients.

Infusion toxicity was also shown to correlate with total nucleated cell (TNC) dose and granulocytes, which have reduced osmotic tolerance and tend to lyse releasing cytokines during cryopreservation (Foïs et al. 2007; Davis et al. 1990). RBCs lyse at thaw, and higher RBC concentration was shown to be associated with cardiac toxicity and arrhythmia (Alessandrino et al. 1999).

Besides DMSO's toxicity to the patient, the same levels of DMSO that help maintain cells during cryopreservation can be lethal to the cells when thawed (Arakawa et al. 1990; Fahy 1986). DMSO destabilizes the phospholipid membranes at higher temperatures, increasing the membrane leakage and cell destruction (Arakawa et al. 1990; Anchordoguy et al. 1992). Therefore, thawing approaches of cryopreserved PB graft should either include steps to minimize the cell exposure time to DMSO or include measures that will remove DMSO rapidly after thaw.

7.4 Thawing Practices

Methods to process cryopreserved PB graft for transplantation should minimize cell loss, maintain cell viability, and prevent introduction of microbial contamination.

Thawing should be done rapidly to avoid the possibility of recrystallization of any small intracellular ice nuclei, and steps should be taken to reduce DMSO concentration to prevent potentially damaging osmotic swelling (Woods et al. 2000).

7.4.1 Bedside Thaw

Direct thaw and administration of a unit to the patient with no additional manipulation are the most commonly used methods for infusion of cryopreserved PB graft for adult patients. It is often called *bedside thaw* because it is typically performed in adjacent to the patient bedside, thus limiting the time between thaw and infusion and reducing the potential damage to the cells from DMSO exposure.

To maintain the product frozen, it is delivered in a validated container. Some centers transport the bags on dry ice that can maintain the temperature between −75 and −80 °C; most transplant centers use liquid nitrogen-charged dry shippers that maintain the temperature below −135 °C. The thawing rate is as important as the cryopreservation rate. Rapid thaw can help reduce intracellular recrystallization of ice due to suboptimal cryopreservation procedure (Mazur 2004; Baust et al. 2009). HPCs are typically cryopreserved with low cooling rate (1 °C/min; see Chap. 6), but it was shown that thawing in 37 °C sustains higher cell viability compared to 4 °C (Bowman et al. 1996). Once ready to be thawed, the cryopreserved bag is removed from the dry shipper and is placed in an additional overwrap to prevent potential leaking in case of compromised bags. The wrapped unit is placed in a water bath containing sterile water validated to maintain temperature ranging between 37 and 40 °C. The unit is removed from the water bath when all the ice crystals dissolve. Many laboratories use alternative dry warming devices, instead of a water bath for thawing. The advantage of these devices is the fact that the units do not have to be submerged in water, a potential source of microbial contamination, and the device cleaning between products is easy.

When a unit is thawed, it has to be administered to the patient promptly to reduce damage to the cells. If multiple units are required for the transplant, they will be thawed sequentially to ensure that the previous unit was infused without adverse reaction. Once thawed as described above, the product can be infused directly from the bag, or it can be transferred to a syringe. Infusion pumps are usually not used, and most centers infuse by gravity. The use of a syringe allows increasing the infusion rate, but transferring the product to a syringe in the noncontrolled environment of the patient bedside does increase the risk of introducing contamination.

Bedside thaw is an easy method that does not require highly trained technologists and can be performed by the nurses in the unit, if trained properly. Additionally, it results in very little cell loss, especially if the empty bag is adequately flushed with saline. It is commonly used in adult patients that can tolerate relatively higher volumes of DMSO compared to children.

The *direct thaw method* carries multiple disadvantages. Larger volumes of DMSO are associated with adverse outcomes, and poorly mobilized autologous patient often have to tolerate large infusion volume to achieve transplant $CD34^+$ cell dose. To reduce the chance of side effects, the maximum recommended dose of DMSO is 1 mL/kg of recipient body weight per 24 h, which can sometimes force infusion over multiple days (AABB et al. 2016). Adverse events were reported for infusion of thawed PB HPCs, some of them severe or even fatal. Once the product is thawed, any delay in infusion can further subject the cells to potential damage due to exposure to relatively high concentration of DMSO, without the benefit of the stabilizing effect of the protein- or colloid-based wash or dilution solution. Additional downside is the fact that infusion preparation occurs outside of the controlled laboratory environment, preventing characterization and confirmation of product cellular content. If samples are obtained at the bedside for retrospective testing, the cell integrity and viability might be compromised due to DMSO exposure by the time they reach the laboratory.

7.4.2 Clumping and the Use of Filter

Delayed infusion of thawed products can result in clumping formation. Granulocyte breakage results in release of toxins and DNA which were shown to result in clumping. Clumping can clog the infusion access line and can pose additional risk to the patient. A 170-μm blood filter can be used to remove these clots and is used by many transplant centers (Alessandrino et al. 1999; López-Jiménez et al. 1994; Kessinger et al. 1990); some centers prefer not to use the filter due to potential HPC lost and blockage of the filter.

7.4.3 Thaw and Wash

The *thawing and washing method* is designed to reduce the volume of DMSO and other elements such as cell debris and cytokines and decrease additional long-term cell damage and potential infusion adverse reaction. There is immediate dilution of the thawed product with a solution containing protein, colloids, or anticoagulant additives. This helps stabilize the membrane and immediately reduces DMSO concentration and is followed by centrifugation step and removal of most of the DMSO and other toxins. Alternatively, automated wash procedures are used.

The wash procedure is performed in the controlled laboratory environment. The wash procedure is based on the method described by Rubinstein and colleagues for preparation of CB unit (Rubinstein et al. 1995). The wash solution described in Rubinstein's report is a mixture of Dextran 40 and HSA. Some laboratories use a similar solution for wash of PB HPC product. Additional solutions are described by others, which are usually an isotonic based buffer, such as saline or Plasmalyte A, combined with additives such as HSA and citrate dextrose (ACD-A) (Foïs et al. 2007; Scerpa et al. 2011; Syme et al. 2004). The wash solution is usually prepared on the day of infusion and maintained refrigerated until processing. The traditional method uses dilution of the product with the wash solution, followed by centrifugation for DMSO and debris removal. The cryopreserved bag is placed in an overwrap and thawed as described above. Multiple bags can be thawed at the same time. The thawed unit is slowly reconstituted with an equal volume wash solution and further diluted with the same solution. The maximal volume depends on the size of the thawed product and the transfer pack that is used. These typically range between 300 and 600 mL. The cells are than centrifuged in 800–1000 × *g* for 10–20 min, usually in 4–10 °C. The supernatant is removed, and the cells are resuspended in the same solution to a final volume that is similar to the original cryopreserved product volume. This procedure removes most of the DMSO.

Unlike *bedside thaw method*, *thawing and washing method* is done in the controlled laboratory environment with all critical steps being performed in the biological safety cabinet, allowing sampling for prospective testing such as viability and potency. The major advantage of the wash procedure is the reduction in adverse reactions rates, probably due to the much lower volume of DMSO infused. Multiple studies have shown significantly lower infusion-related adverse effect of washed PB graft compared to non-washed, across all types of side effects monitored (Syme et al. 2004; Sánchez-Salinas et al. 2012; Akkök et al. 2009). This method was proven to reduce DMSO osmotic damage and maintain cell viability. When compared to the *bedside thaw method*, cell viability is stable for many hours, providing longer expiration time (Rodríguez et al. 2005).

Despite all the benefits listed above, the *thaw and wash* procedure does carry some disadvantages. The wash and centrifugation steps are associated with progenitor cell loss. Comparison studies report an average of 20% loss of TNC count post-wash and a similar loss of $CD34^+$ cells (Syme et al. 2004; Akkök et al. 2009). Some of these cells can be recovered by applying a second centrifugation step, but this will increase the processing time and exposes the cells to additional damage. Akokke and colleagues showed that although time to neutrophil engraftment was similar for washed and non-washed autologous products, platelet engraftment was significantly delayed for washed products, resulting in a significantly higher number of platelet transfusions for patients (Akkök et al. 2009). Another factor to be considered when choosing to use the *wash procedure* is the risk of bag breakage. Although bag integrity can be compromised due to inappropriate bag sealing or during cryopreservation, the risk of bag breakage increases with any additional processing step, such as centrifugation. Compromised bag can result in major cell loss and potential microbial contamination. Lastly, it is also important to note that the *thaw and wash method* does require the availability of highly trained and qualified laboratory technologists, and for small programs that perform few transplants per year, this can be challenging.

7.5 Expert Point of View

In order to determine how to prepare PB HPCs for infusion, transplant centers need to assess multiple factors including the transplant program setting, the patient demographics, and the availability of trained laboratory staff. By reviewing these factors and the pros and cons of each method, programs can perform a risk assessment and come up with the best fitting approach.

Bedside thaw method is probably the most commonly used method for infusion of previously cryopreserved PB HPCs and, if done properly, results most of the time in hematological reconstitution. But many studies have shown that direct infusion of previously cryopreserved PB HPCs results in occurrence of adverse events, mostly mild or moderate. Most of these adverse events are attributed to the presence of DMSO, which has dose-dependent toxicity (López-Jiménez et al. 1994; Kessinger et al. 1990; Rowley et al. 1999). Factors such as TNC dose and granulocytes concentration are also shown to correlate with thawed autologous PB-mobilized HPC infusion adverse events (Cordoba et al. 2007; Khera et al. 2012).

Despite the relatively higher rates of adverse events, small volume adult transplant programs with limited availability of highly trained laboratory staff, or programs that do not have processing laboratory on site and use outside services, should consider using the *bedside thaw method*. The method does not reduce the DMSO volume, or any other toxins, but is simple and requires no processing.

On the other hand, programs that serve pediatric patient population or high-risk patients (see text above) might consider using the *thaw wash method* to reduce DMSO toxicity. The main disadvantages of the latter method is the complexity of the process and the risk of cell loss, but most comparison studies have shown no differences in neutrophil and platelet engraftment time between the methods, and sometimes the *wash method* results in a slightly shorter engraftment time, probably due to higher cell viability. All studies comparing infusion side effect outcomes demonstrate significantly lower rates for the washed products. This is the main reason to use the wash procedure, especially when serving very frail or pediatric patient population. This method removes most of the DMSO and other toxins and sustains cell viability for extended time.

7.6 Future Direction

Future efforts should be directed to improve and standardize cell/graft manufacturing, cryopreservation, and thawing of hematopoietic graft. Better understanding of the mechanism of cell damage by cryopreservation will help optimize the process. That should include parameters such as sample harvest and preparation, optimal cell concentration, additives used in the process, freezing curves, and more. Additionally, development of alternative, less toxic cryoprotectant agents will reduce the need to wash cells and will result in more stable products with lower toxicity.

There are constantly ongoing attempts to develop alternative cryoprotecting molecules either without or with reduced DMSO concentration (Bakken et al. 2003; Zeisberger et al. 2011). Disaccharide molecules such as trehalose and sucrose were shown to maintain membrane and protein integrity during cryopreservation, and their combination with DMSO concentration as low as 2.5% in cryopreservation of CB was shown to be compatible with the traditional 10% DMSO concentration (Woods et al. 2000; Rodrigues et al. 2008; Zhang et al. 2003). Recent publication by Svalgaard and colleagues explored the use of low-molecular-weight carbohydrate Pentaisomaltose (PIM) as an alternative to DMSO in cryopreservation of PB grafts. They demonstrated that progenitor cell recovery and potency were similar between PB products cryopreserved with PIM and DMSO (Svalgaard et al. 2016).

Automated wash devices are available for many years but are not often used by processing facility for PB HPC wash. They are expensive, require additional training, and are associated with the risk of additional HPC loss. Few automated devices were evaluated for washing of cryopreserved HPC products. Automated washing systems can provide a uniform standardized method that, if done properly, can increase cell recovery and reduce potential introduction of microbial contamination during processing. Some of these are 510(k) devices licensed for a specific use, and others have more usage flexibility. Regardless, each device has to be validated for the specific cell source use. Different automated devices were shown by few groups to result in high cell recovery and viable progenitor cells (Foïs et al.

2007; Scerpa et al. 2011; Sánchez-Salinas et al. 2012; Rodríguez et al. 2005; Perotti et al. 2004). All systems apply a single-use disposable set and different cell separation methodology. They were all shown to remove most of the DMSO and result in high CD34⁺ cell recovery. TNC recovery with these systems is usually between 75% and 90%, probably due to removal of granulocytes that do not sustain the cryopreservation and thawing process. Fois and colleagues used the traditional COBE 2991 cell washer, which uses centrifugal force to separate cells based on their type, size, and density, to wash cryopreserved PB HPCs. They reported substantial TNC loss, mainly due to granulocyte presence, and high CD34⁺ cell recovery. Few groups demonstrated the use of SEPAX cell processing system (Biosafe, Switzerland), a device designed as CB processing system, for washing of PB HPCs. This device separates cellular components through rotation of the syringe chamber and component transfer through a syringe piston. The wash with SEPAX proves to be at least as good as the *manual wash method* (see text above) and results in high CD34⁺ cell recovery (Scerpa et al. 2011; Sánchez-Salinas et al. 2012), CytoMate (Baxter, Chicago, IL), a spinning membrane against cell separating device, was shown to remove more than 95% of DMSO from products and recover more than 80% of CD34⁺ cells. The products resulted in significantly lower rates of infusion adverse reactions, and as demonstrated for washed products, time to neutrophil platelet engraftment was compatible to non-washed products, regardless of the TNC loss (Rodríguez et al. 2005; Calmels et al. 2003; Lemarie et al. 2005). Few other devices, such as the Lovo Cell Processing System (Fresenius Kabi), were introduced in the last few years. The expansion of the cellular therapy field and the introduction of new therapies encourage the industry to manufacture smaller and better applications for cell processing that are also in compliance with good manufacturing practices (GMPs).

References

AABB AAoTB, American Red Cross, American Society for Blood and Marrow, Transplantation ASfA, America's Blood Centers, College of American Pathologists, Cord Blood Association, Foundation for the Accreditation of, Cellular Therapy I, International NetCord Foundation, International Society for Cellular Therapy, JACIE Accreditation Office, Program NMD (2016) Circular of information for the use of cellular therapy products. Bethesda, MD, AABB

Akkök CA, Holte MR, Tangen JM, Ostenstad B, Bruserud O (2009) Hematopoietic engraftment of dimethyl sulfoxide-depleted autologous peripheral blood progenitor cells. Transfusion 49(2):354–361

Alessandrino P, Bernasconi P, Caldera D et al (1999) Adverse events occurring during bone marrow or peripheral blood progenitor cell infusion: analysis of 126 cases. Bone Marrow Transplant 23(6):533–537

Anchordoguy TJ, Carpenter JF, Crowe JH, Crowe LM (1992) Temperature-dependent perturbation of phospholipid bilayers by dimethylsulfoxide. Biochim Biophys Acta 1104(1):117–122

Arakawa T, Carpenter JF, Kita YA, Crowe JH (1990) The basis for toxicity of certain cryoprotectants: a hypothesis. Cryobiology 27:401–415

Bakken AM, Bruserud O, Abrahamsen JF (2003) No differences in colony formation of peripheral blood stem cells frozen with 5% or 10% dimethyl sulfoxide. J Hematother Stem Cell Res 12(3):351–358

Baust JG, Gao D, Baust JM (2009) Cryopreservation: an emerging paradigm change. Organogenesis 5(3):90–96

Benekli M, Anderson B, Wentling D, Bernstein S, Czuczman M, McCarthy P (2000) Severe respiratory depression after dimethylsulphoxide-containing autologous stem cell infusion in a patient with AL amyloidosis. Bone Marrow Transplant 25(12):1299–1301

Bothner U, Georgieff M, Vogt NH (1998) Assessment of the safety and tolerance of 6% hydroxyethyl starch (200/0.5) solution: a randomized, controlled epidemiology study. Anesth Analg 86(4):850–855

Bowman CA, Yu M, Cottler-Fox M (1996) Evaluation of methods for preparing and thawing cryopreserved CD34+ and CD34− cell lines for use as reagents in flow cytometry of hematopoietic progenitor cells. Transfusion 36(11-12):985–988

Brave M, Farrell A, Ching Lin S et al (2010) FDA review summary: Mozobil in combination with granulocyte colony-stimulating factor to mobilize hematopoietic stem cells to the peripheral blood for collection and subsequent autologous transplantation. Oncology 78(3-4):282–288

Broxmeyer HE, Srour EF, Hangoc G, Cooper S, Anderson SA, Bodine DM (2003) High-efficiency recovery of functional hematopoietic progenitor and stem cells from human cord blood cryopreserved for 15 years. Proc Natl Acad Sci U S A 100(2):645–650

Calmels B, Houzé P, Hengesse JC, Ducrot T, Malenfant C, Chabannon C (2003) Preclinical evaluation of an automated closed fluid management device: Cytomate, for washing out DMSO from hematopoietic stem cell grafts after thawing. Bone Marrow Transplant 31(9):823–828

Cordoba R, Arrieta R, Kerguelen A, Hernandez-Navarro F (2007) The occurrence of adverse events during the infusion of autologous peripheral blood stem cells is related to the number of granulocytes in the leukapheresis product. Bone Marrow Transplant 40(11):1063–1067

Davis JM, Rowley SD, Braine HG, Piantadosi S, Santos GW (1990) Clinical toxicity of cryopreserved bone marrow graft infusion. Blood 75(3):781–786

Dhodapkar M, Goldberg SL, Tefferi A, Gertz MA (1994) Reversible encephalopathy after cryopreserved peripheral blood stem cell infusion. Am J Hematol 45(2):187–188

Donnenberg AD, Koch EK, Griffin DL et al (2002) Viability of cryopreserved BM progenitor cells stored for more than a decade. Cytotherapy 4(2):157–163

Fahy GM (1986) The relevance of cryoprotectant "toxicity" to cryobiology. Cryobiology 23(1):1–13

Foïs E, Desmartin M, Benhamida S et al (2007) Recovery, viability and clinical toxicity of thawed and washed haematopoietic progenitor cells: analysis of 952 autologous peripheral blood stem cell transplantations. Bone Marrow Transplant 40(9):831–835

Hoyt R, Szer J, Grigg A (2000) Neurological events associated with the infusion of cryopreserved bone marrow and/or peripheral blood progenitor cells. Bone Marrow Transplant 25(12):1285–1287

Kao GS (2009) Assessment of collection quality. In: Areman EM, Loper K (eds) Cellular therapy: principles, methods, and regulations. AABB, Bethesda, MD, pp 291–302

Keating GM (2011) Plerixafor: a review of its use in stem-cell mobilization in patients with lymphoma or multiple myeloma. Drugs 71(12):1623–1647

Kessinger A, Schmit-Pokorny K, Smith D, Armitage J (1990) Cryopreservation and infusion of autologous peripheral blood stem cells. Bone Marrow Transplant 5(Suppl 1):25–27

Khera N, Jinneman J, Storer BE et al (2012) Limiting the daily total nucleated cell dose of cryopreserved peripheral blood stem cell products for autologous transplantation improves infusion-related safety with no adverse impact on hematopoietic engraftment. Biol Blood Marrow Transplant 18(2):220–228

Lemarie C, Calmels B, Malenfant C et al (2005) Clinical experience with the delivery of thawed and washed autologous blood cells, with an automated closed fluid management device: CytoMate. Transfusion 45(5):737–742

López-Jiménez J, Cerveró C, Muñoz A et al (1994) Cardiovascular toxicities related to the infusion of cryopreserved grafts: results of a controlled study. Bone Marrow Transplant 13(6):789–793

Lovelock JE, Bishop MW (1959) Prevention of freezing damage to living cells by dimethyl sulphoxide. Nature 183(4672):1394–1395

Mazur P (2004) Principles of cryobiology. In: Fuller BJ, Lane N, Benson E (eds) Life in the frozen state. CRC, Boca Raton, FL, pp 3–66

Mazur P, Leibo SP, Chu EH (1972) A two-factor hypothesis of freezing injury. Evidence from Chinese hamster tissue-culture cells. Exp Cell Res 71(2):345–355

Pagano MB, Harmon C, Cooling L et al (2016) Use of hydroxyethyl starch in leukocytapheresis procedures does not increase renal toxicity. Transfusion 56(11):2848–2856

Pasquini M, Zhu X (2015) Current uses and outcomes of hematopoietic stem cell transplantation: CIBMTR summary slides. http://www.cibmtr.org

Perotti CG, Del Fante C, Viarengo G et al (2004) A new automated cell washer device for thawed cord blood units. Transfusion 44(6):900–906

Rapoport AP, Rowe JM, Packman CH, Ginsberg SJ (1991) Cardiac arrest after autologous marrow infusion. Bone Marrow Transplant 7(5):401–403

Rodrigues JP, Paraguassú-Braga FH, Carvalho L, Abdelhay E, Bouzas LF, Porto LC (2008) Evaluation of trehalose and sucrose as cryoprotectants for hematopoietic stem cells of umbilical cord blood. Cryobiology 56(2):144–151

Rodríguez L, Velasco B, García J, Martín-Henao GA (2005) Evaluation of an automated cell processing device to reduce the dimethyl sulfoxide from hematopoietic grafts after thawing. Transfusion 45(8):1391–1397

Rowley S, MacLeod B, Heimfeld S, Holmberg L, Bensinger W (1999) Severe central nervous system toxicity associated with the infusion of cryopreserved PBSC components. Cytotherapy 1(4):311–317

Rubinstein P, Dobrila L, Rosenfield RE et al (1995) Processing and cryopreservation of placental/umbilical cord blood for unrelated bone marrow reconstitution. Proc Natl Acad Sci U S A 92(22):10119–10122

Runckel DN, Swanson JR (1980) Effect of dimethyl sulfoxide on serum osmolality. Clin Chem 26(12):1745–1747

Samoszuk M, Reid ME, Toy PT (1983) Intravenous dimethylsulfoxide therapy causes severe hemolysis mimicking a hemolytic transfusion reaction. Transfusion 23(5):405

Sánchez-Salinas A, Cabañas-Perianes V, Blanquer M et al (2012) An automatic wash method for dimethyl sulfoxide removal in autologous hematopoietic stem cell transplantation decreases the adverse effects related to infusion. Transfusion 52(11):2382–2386

Sauer-Heilborn A, Kadidlo D, McCullough J (2004) Patient care during infusion of hematopoietic progenitor cells. Transfusion 44(6):907–916

Scerpa MC, Daniele N, Landi F et al (2011) Automated washing of human progenitor cells: evaluation of apoptosis and cell necrosis. Transfus Med 21(6):402–407

Smith DM, Weisenburger DD, Bierman P, Kessinger A, Vaughan WP, Armitage JO (1987) Acute renal failure associated with autologous bone marrow transplantation. Bone Marrow Transplant 2(2):195–201

Snyder EL, Haley NR (eds) (2004) Cellular therapy: a physician's handbook, 1st edn. Bethesda, MD, AABB

Spurr EE, Wiggins NE, Marsden KA, Lowenthal RM, Ragg SJ (2002) Cryopreserved human haematopoietic stem cells retain engraftment potential after extended (5-14 years) cryostorage. Cryobiology 44(3):210–217

Svalgaard JD, Haastrup EK, Reckzeh K et al (2016) Low-molecular-weight carbohydrate Pentaisomaltose may replace dimethyl sulfoxide as a safer cryoprotectant for cryopreservation of peripheral blood stem cells. Transfusion 56(5):1088–1095

Syme R, Bewick M, Stewart D, Porter K, Chadderton T, Glück S (2004) The role of depletion of dimethyl sulfoxide before autografting: on hematologic recovery, side effects, and toxicity. Biol Blood Marrow Transplant 10(2):135–141

Vercueil A, Grocott MP, Mythen MG (2005) Physiology, pharmacology, and rationale for colloid administration for the maintenance of effective hemodynamic stability in critically ill patients. Transfus Med Rev 19(2):93–109

Wagner JE, Barker JN, DeFor TE et al (2002) Transplantation of unrelated donor umbilical cord blood in 102 patients with malignant and nonmalignant diseases: influence of CD34 cell dose and HLA disparity on treatment-related mortality and survival. Blood 100(5):1611–1618

Windrum P, Morris TC, Drake MB, Niederwieser D, Ruutu T, Subcommittee ECLWPC (2005) Variation in dimethyl sulfoxide use in stem cell transplantation: a survey of EBMT centres. Bone Marrow Transplant 36(7):601–603

Woods EJ, Liu J, Derrow CW, Smith FO, Williams DA, Critser JK (2000) Osmometric and permeability characteristics of human placental/umbilical cord blood CD34+ cells and their application to cryopreservation. J Hematother Stem Cell Res 9(2):161–173

Yellowlees P, Greenfield C, McIntyre N (1980) Dimethylsulphoxide-induced toxicity. Lancet 2(8202):1004–1006

Zambelli A, Poggi G, Da Prada G et al (1998) Clinical toxicity of cryopreserved circulating progenitor cells infusion. Anticancer Res 18(6B):4705–4708

Zeisberger SM, Schulz JC, Mairhofer M et al (2011) Biological and physicochemical characterization of a serum- and xeno-free chemically defined cryopreservation procedure for adult human progenitor cells. Cell Transplant 20(8):1241–1257

Zenhäusern R, Tobler A, Leoncini L, Hess OM, Ferrari P (2000) Fatal cardiac arrhythmia after infusion of dimethyl sulfoxide-cryopreserved hematopoietic stem cells in a patient with severe primary cardiac amyloidosis and end-stage renal failure. Ann Hematol 79(9):523–526

Zhang XB, Li K, Yau KH et al (2003) Trehalose ameliorates the cryopreservation of cord blood in a preclinical system and increases the recovery of CFUs, long-term culture-initiating cells, and nonobese diabetic-SCID repopulating cells. Transfusion 43(2):265–272

Part 2

HPC, Cord Blood

Cord Blood Donor Qualification

8

Ngaire J. Elwood

8.1 Introduction

Cord blood (CB) donor qualification is an active process to determine suitability and safety of a CB unit (CBU) for clinical use. In the context of hematopoietic cell transplantation (HCT), the CBU must be suitable and safe to provide long-term hematopoietic reconstitution posttransplantation. The hematopoietic CD34$^+$ cells contained within a CBU must be able to engraft post-infusion into the bone marrow niche in order to self-renew, proliferate, and differentiate into all lineages of the hematopoietic compartment to restore hematopoiesis. Therefore, the CD34$^+$ cells must engraft and result in successful patient outcome and the CB must not transmit infectious disease or genetic abnormalities.

The CB donor is the newborn baby. Consent on behalf of the donor is given by the mother (and sometimes father), who is considered a "surrogate". Sometimes, for clarity of documentation, the delineation of CB donor may be broken down to "infant donor" or "maternal donor." An infant donor is a newborn from whose placenta or umbilical cord the CBU is obtained. A maternal donor is the mother who carries the infant donor to delivery (FACT 2016). This may be the genetic or surrogate mother; knowledge of which is important for donor qualification.

In contrast to other types of hematopoietic progenitor cell (HPC) donors, where the cells are usually used within a short time of the donation, a CBU donation is stored long term. Therefore, there is the potential to perform follow-up medical history of mother and donor (infant) and repeat infectious disease testing on the

N.J. Elwood, Ph.D.
BMDI Cord Blood Bank, Murdoch Children's Research Institute, The Royal Children's Hospital, Parkville, VIC, Australia

Department of Paediatrics, University of Melbourne, Parkville, VIC, Australia
e-mail: ngaire.elwood@mcri.edu.au

J. Schwartz, B.H. Shaz (eds.), *Best Practices in Processing and Storage for Hematopoietic Cell Transplantation*, Advances and Controversies in Hematopoietic Transplantation and Cell Therapy,
https://doi.org/10.1007/978-3-319-58949-7_8

mother, if desired. This potential is to be maximized for CBU donor qualification. The majority of unrelated CB banks (CBBs) around the world collect, process, and store CB for the purposes of unrelated CB transplants (CBT). CBU donor qualification is therefore vital prior to long-term storage, as these products may be stored for many years before they are released to patients. The content of this chapter is directed toward CBU donor qualification for unrelated CBBs, but it is also relevant for those CBBs storing family or related CB units for CBT. The degree of qualification and the acceptable minimum criteria may not need to be as stringent within the family CBB setting due to autologous or directed use of these CBU.

The parameters that can and should be considered for CBU donor qualification include quality, infectious disease screening, and genetic risks. Steps include donor history questionnaire, genetic screening, and infectious disease testing and product quality assessment.

8.2 Cord Blood Donor Qualification Process

8.2.1 Recruitment of Potential Donors

The CB donor selection commences with an expectant mother deciding to donate her infant's CB to a CBB. Sometimes this decision might be the result of a mother proactively investigating CBU donation options but more often is a result of targeted recruitment by the CBB. This may be in the form of brochures or information provided during antenatal care, may be a conversation with an obstetrician or midwife, or may be via active recruitment at the time of delivery.

8.2.2 Informed Consent

Prior to the collection and processing of CB, informed consent must be obtained from the maternal donor (and in some CBBs also the other partner with parental responsibilities) for the CBU to be collected, processed, tested, stored, and administered for CBT and potentially for research. A CBU will only be acceptable for banking and distribution if appropriate informed consent has been obtained. In the case of family banking, this consent may be in the form of an agreement between the CBB and the family. For unrelated CBB, the information provided to potential donors and the consent process will have been approved by an appropriate Institutional Review Board (IRB) or Human Ethics Committee and must comply with applicable law relevant to that country and any published code of practice on consent. The "informed consent" procedures should be designed to protect the interests of the infant donor's family and educate the maternal donor about the various options for CBU use. Furthermore, it is important that the "informed consent" or an agreement between the mother and the CBB is obtained and documented while the mother is able to concentrate on the information and is not distracted by the labor during the process. Thus, some CBBs will use "mini-consent" or "consent for collection only" if the mother is progressed in labor, with a full consent being obtained after delivery but before any processing of the collected CBU takes place. CBU donor qualification must ensure that an approved consent or agreement process is in place and that appropriate informed consent has been obtained for the CBU collection, processing, testing, storage, and use.

8.2.3 Donor History Questionnaire

CBU collection starts with the recruitment and screening of potential donors, usually by ensuring up-front such expectant mothers who would like to be CBU donors and meet requirements similar to those set by AABB's hematopoietic progenitor cell, CB donor history questionnaire. Prior to, or following, the successful collection of CBU, the maternal donor will be asked to complete the donor history questionnaire relating to parental and family health, travel, obstetric, and delivery history. Since the only way that the CBU could be exposed to infectious disease is via the placenta while in utero, maternal blood is used as the surrogate to screen for infectious disease markers.

When a potential maternal donor indicates an interest in donating CBU to an unrelated bank or sometimes soon after they have provided consent for CBU collection and had the CBU collected, an initial screening is undertaken to exclude donors whose CBU may provide a potential risk for transmission of diseases such as hepatitis B and C, HIV-1 and HIV-2 (AIDS), syphilis, and HTLV-I and HTLV-II. CBBs require that the maternal donor complete a CB donor history questionnaire (DHQ), where key questions are asked to identify risk factors for infectious diseases that can be transmitted by transfusion. The types of questions asked are sensitive and personal (Table 8.1), but questions should be answered accurately. Through asking such questions, it is often possible to exclude high-risk donors at this early stage of the donation process, thereby saving time, resources, and money from going through with the collection process or, if the CB has already been collected, from processing, testing, and storing the unit long term.

Every CBB will have written criteria against which the mother and infant are evaluated in terms of their eligibility as a CB donor. Accrediting bodies, such as the Foundation for the Accreditation of Cellular Therapy (FACT), do not define an acceptable donor but instead require that the CBB define its own specifications for CBU banking. Many CBB will use the criteria outlined by their local authorities (e.g., FDA) or will use the guidelines to develop guidelines specific to CB. Ideally these guidelines will provide the acceptable answers to questions that are asked in a comprehensive maternal and family history questionnaire, which includes questions regarding travel and infant donor birth details, and then provide guidance as to how to manage answers that are unacceptable for that CB to be stored for banking or used for CBT. The guidelines used to evaluate the answers to the questions are beyond the scope of this chapter but should reference each disease or issue and provide guidance as to whether to accept or reject the CB.

Table 8.1 Cord blood donor history questionnaire example (Source: AusCord Donor Declaration)

To the best of your knowledge have you	
1.	Ever thought you could be infected with HIV or have AIDS?
2.	Used drugs by injection or been injected, even once, with drugs not prescribed by a doctor or dentist in the past 5 years?
3.	Ever had treatment with clotting factors such as Factor VIII or Factor IX?
4.	Ever had a test that showed you had hepatitis B and C and HIV or HTLV?
5.	Received a blood transfusion or injection of blood or blood products (red cells, Platelets, granulocytes, or plasma) in
5a.	The United Kingdom (i.e., England, Scotland, Wales, Northern Ireland, the Channel Islands, Isle of Man, Gibraltar, and the Falkland Islands) or France **after 1 January 1980**?
5b.	Central/South America or Mexico **ever**?
In the last 12 months have you	
6.	Had an illness with swollen glands with a rash, with or without a fever?
7.	Engaged in sexual activity with someone you think would answer "yes" to any of questions 1–6?
8.	Engaged in sexual activity with a **new partner** (less than 12 months ago) who currently lives or has previously lived overseas?
9.	Engaged in sexual activity with a male who you think might be bisexual?
10.	Been a sex worker (e.g., received payment for sex in money, gifts, or drugs)?
11.	Engaged in sexual activity with a male or female sex worker?
12.	Been imprisoned in a prison or lock-up?
13.	Had (yellow) jaundice or hepatitis or been living with, or had sex with, someone who has?
During pregnancy have you	
14.	Been injured with a used needle (needlestick injury)?
15.	Had someone else's blood or body fluid splash to your eyes, mouth, nose, or to a broken skin?
16.	Had a tattoo (including cosmetic tattooing), skin piercing, electrolysis, or acupuncture?
17.	Had a blood transfusion or injection of blood or blood products (red cells, platelets, granulocytes, or plasma), including an intrauterine transfusion?

Maternal and infant donor evaluation and management are critical components of CB donor qualification.

8.2.3.1 Family Medical and Genetic History

A maternal history is taken to identify infectious or genetic disease in the mother that may affect the HPCs of the fetus, either by placental transfer or by genetic inheritance. Key questions are asked of the mother in order to cover the full scope of potential medical issues, which can then be delved into should a positive answer be given. A detailed family medical and genetic history with specific questioning is crucial. A range of medical and genetic diseases can be transmitted from either parent to the fetus and, if affecting the hematopoietic lineage, be passed on through the donor to a recipient of the CB. Thus, the history must document all diseases that occur in the family and must include family on both the maternal and paternal side. It is important to have documented history of problems in parents, children, grandparents, aunts, uncles, and cousins. Some diseases may not be apparent in the newborn until after 6 months of age, and hence, where possible, a CBB should impress on mothers the importance of remaining in touch and informing the CBB of changes in the health of the infant. In assessing CB donor qualification, it is also important to ask questions about the family ethnic background. Some genetic diseases are more prevalent in specific racial groups, e.g., sickle cell disease in African, African-American, and Middle Eastern individuals; thalassemia in individuals from Mediterranean and Asian countries; and rare, recessively inherited metabolic diseases and immunodeficiency disorders in racial groups where consanguinity has been common.

8.2.3.2 Obstetric History

The CB donor qualification assessment should also include a full review of obstetric history (for both for pregnancy and delivery). The prime risk during pregnancy relates to exposure to infections and to medications, where the importance of most medications is the disease for which they were given. As part of the CB donor qualification assessment, it is important to identify that the infant donor is healthy and well at the time of birth and thereafter. Labor and delivery information, as well as physical assessment of the mother and baby, is documented as part of donor qualification. Physical or laboratory abnormalities identified at birth may, apart from leading to exclusion of the CB, reflect a disease in the newborn baby. An illness in the perinatal period may indicate that the CB is not suitable for use.

8.2.3.3 Travel History

A maternal travel/residency history is an important aspect of CB donor qualification. Certain countries have an increased frequency of infectious diseases (such as HIV, Chagas disease, Ebola virus, Zika virus, and malaria). If the mother is infected, this disease may be transmitted via the placenta to the fetus. It is important for the CBB to record details of country of travel/residency, as well as year(s) of residency and duration of stay, that can then be assessed to determine CB donor qualification. Each CBB will usually refer to a table or document (often based on the local blood authority guidelines in their country) that classifies countries and regions for the purpose of assessing possible maternal risk, highlighting which infectious diseases may be of concern or endemic in a particular country. Donors with a possible risk of acquiring these diseases are not necessarily excluded from being CB donors, but rather this knowledge allows appropriate infectious disease screening that is pertinent to the area of travel/residency (e.g., malaria antibody screening). Table 8.2 lists some of the infectious diseases that are of concern when assessing a travel/residency history (Source: AusCord Guide to selection of mothers and donors). The list of relevant countries or regions will be updated from time to time, dependent of outbreaks of transmittable disease in new regions or countries.

Table 8.2 Infectious diseases of concern when assessing a travel/residency history

HIV	Pertains to the risk of sexually acquired HIV infection in donors with *new sexual partners* who have resided in those areas. Examples of countries of risk: Botswana, Cambodia, Congo
Chagas	Mothers who were born in or transfused in these areas could have chronic Chagas infection without symptoms. Examples of countries of risk: Argentina, Belize, Honduras
Ebola/Marburg	Endemic in some countries in Africa. Examples of countries of risk: Angola, Congo, Kenya
Malaria	Mothers who have travelled or resided in these areas could have malaria without displaying symptoms for some time. Examples of countries of risk: Afghanistan, Indonesia, Papua New Guinea
Dengue and chikungunya	There are countries or regions where outbreaks of either of these two very similar arboviruses are known to occur but where no malaria restriction applies. Examples of countries of risk: Martinique, Dominica, Singapore
West Nile virus	Historically endemic to a number of countries in Africa, Asia, and the Middle East. A virulent strain emerged in 1999 in North America. Examples of countries of risk: the United States, Saint Pierre and Miquelon, Canada
Schistosomiasis (also known as bilharzia)	Endemic in some countries. Mothers who have travelled or resided in these areas may have a past history of bilharziasis. Examples of countries of risk: Iraq, Jamaica, Saudi Arabia
Rabies	Most countries, including many developed areas like North America, continue to report rabies transmission. Mothers who have suffered *an animal bite or scratch* in these areas may have infection without symptoms and/or have received rabies immunoglobulin from an overseas source. Examples of countries of risk: Bangladesh, France, the Philippines
Zika virus	This virus, first identified in 1947 but confined to Africa and Asia until 2007, is transmitted to humans principally by the *Aedes* mosquitoes, but sexual transmission has been documented from infected males to females. An outbreak was identified in Brazil in early 2015, and more than 34 countries and territories have now reported active transmission

8.3 Donor Testing

8.3.1 Infectious Disease Marker (IDM) Testing Profile

To determine the infectious disease status of CB donors, samples of the maternal blood are collected for the purpose of infectious disease screening. The maternal blood samples serve as a surrogate for the CB unit, and testing should reflect the health of the mother at the time the unit is collected, ideally having been collected within 7 days of CB collection. Testing of maternal blood samples also needs to take into account any factors that may cause plasma dilution that may alter serology test results, such as large-volume infusions of blood or crystalloids prior to collection. Depending upon the country of the CBB, these IDM tests may utilize FDA-approved,

EC-marked, in vitro diagnostic device (IVD)-registered testing kits or some other licensure or registration required by applicable law. Although regulatory authorities and accrediting bodies around the world differ in the infectious disease marker testing mandated by each body and country, there appears to be consensus that all CBUs must be tested for HIV-1/2, HCV, syphilis, and HTLV-I/II antibodies, HBs antigen, HIV-1 nucleic acid amplification technique (NAT), and HCV NAT. Most CBBs also require anti-HBc antibody testing and HBV NAT. Additional testing may be required depending on the donor's history and the characteristics of the cells donated (e.g., malaria, West Nile virus, CMV, Chagas disease, toxoplasma, EBV) and may include emergent disease testing depending on travel history and disease outbreaks (e.g., dengue fever and Zika virus). The results of the IDM tests performed will be evaluated by the CBB prior to the CBU being listed on the cord blood registries and are evaluated by both the CBB and requesting transplant program prior to release.

8.3.2 Microbiological Testing

CBU collection and processing are undertaken using validated aseptic techniques. While the nature of the environment in which CB is procured is such that genital and gastrointestinal microorganisms are prevalent, the cleaning of the cord and procedures for CBU collection should be validated and carried out by sufficiently trained and experienced collection personnel such that the microbial contamination is minimized. Once inside the collection bag, ideally, the CB will be processed within a closed system, with samples removed for testing and addition of cryoprotectant handled in accordance with current good manufacturing practices (cGMP) requirements. It is imperative for unrelated CBU qualification that sterility of the final product is confirmed. However, it is often acceptable for CB units stored for related/autologous use to test positive for microbial contamination, as long as the contaminating microorganism is known and antibiotic drug sensitivity confirmed prior to infusion of the unit. Screening includes aerobic and anaerobic bacteria and fungi, using validated testing methods. Microbial testing validation will have confirmed that the samples and the testing method used will detect the range of commonly observed and expected microorganisms. Often the organisms that are to be tested for are prescribed by applicable law, for example, in accordance with those prescribed in the British Pharmacopoeia. Consideration must also be given to the fact that many mothers are given prophylactic antibiotics at the time of delivery, thereby impacting upon the ability to accurately detect microbial contamination in the CBU. Any microbial-contaminated CBU in an unrelated CBB should be discarded in order to reduce the risk of cross-contamination during long-term cryostorage and avoid the risk of recipient contamination.

8.3.3 Hemoglobinopathy Screening

In the United States, universal newborn screening (NBS) for sickle cell disease (SCD) and other hemoglobinopathies has been performed since 2006 (CDC 2015).

Hemoglobinopathy testing on newborns is not routinely undertaken in most other countries, unless there is a family history of one of the hemoglobinopathies or a genetic risk based on ethnicity. At a minimum, all CBUs banked for unrelated use should be screened for sickle cell disease (SCD) or thalassemia through the maternal and family history questionnaire, and also if ethnicity suggests there may be a higher risk. If not performed on the infant donor at birth, all CBUs released for unrelated use should undergo hemoglobinopathy testing prior to release, using one of the appropriate diagnostic tests, such as isoelectric focusing, high-performance liquid chromatography (HPLC), or molecular methods, in an appropriately accredited testing laboratory. Information relating to hemoglobinopathy risk may also be required in the related CBU setting.

8.4 CBU Quality

As part of the CBU qualification, checks will be made as to the quality of the CBU, both pre- and post-processing. Each CBB will have established criteria for processing and banking of a CBU, with the aim of ensuring the product is acceptable for clinical use. This means the product must be safe and efficacious; there must be enough cells to engraft a recipient; the cells must be viable and show potency. A product must meet all the requirements of safety, quality, identity, potency, and purity, also referred to as SQuIPP (Hillyer 2007; Quinley 2013).

8.4.1 Pre-processing Quality

The volume of CBU collected provides an estimate of the total number of cells that will be present. CBBs have criteria for the minimum acceptable volume of collected CBU that will be taken for processing; this criterion is usually less stringent for family CBB than unrelated CBB, where the intent for unrelated CBB is to bank CBU with a high number of total nucleated cells (TNC), as these will be the more desirable units for CBT. The training and experience of the CBU collector will often impact upon the volumes obtained, but factors such as delayed cord clamping will also impact the volume obtained; the longer the time between delivery and clamping of the cord, the less volume obtained. The mode of CBU collection will also impact upon the volumes obtained; in general higher volumes are obtained with in utero collections compared to ex utero collections (Solves et al. 2003). Both the storage of the CBU at the collection site and the transport from the collection site to the processing facility should be monitored and confirmed to have remained within a validated temperature range to maintain viability and potency of the cells. Upon receipt by the processing laboratory, the CBU will be assessed and should be free of large clots, with the TNC count of sufficient number to meet the minimum criteria for processing. The time between collection and processing must be recorded and confirmed to have occurred within a validated time frame. For unrelated CBUs this ideally should occur within 48 h to ensure the best maintenance of viability and potency (Hubel et al. 2003; Kurtzberg et al. 2005). Longer time periods (e.g., up to 72 h) are often acceptable for related CBUs, where a potentially compromised viability is balanced against the opportunity to bank a family CBU.

8.4.2 Post-processing Quality

Whatever the processing platform used, minimum acceptable criteria, should be achieved with respect to post-processing TNC recovery, cell viability, TNC number, and $CD34^+$ cell number and viability. The sixth edition of the NetCord-FACT Standards for CBB now defines the minimum acceptance criteria for pre- and post-processing parameters (FACT 2016). Each CBB will have established its own minimum criteria for processing and banking, taking into account local economic and operational factors; CB donor qualification is not always based on quality parameters alone.

8.5 Expert Point of View

The fact that CB is a biological product that is collected, processed, and banked for long-term use increases the complexity of donor qualification. Adding to this complexity is the fact that as new tests are developed and introduced over time, it may not be possible to perform these tests on units that are already banked; there may need to be a mechanism to "grandfather" in CBU in the inventory that was banked prior to the new test being available. Donor qualification commences with the recruitment and selection of a suitable maternal donor. Product qualification involves infectious disease monitoring, microbiological testing, and performance of tests to assess cell number, viability, and potency. There are factors that may affect CBU quantity, quality, and potency that are beyond the control of the CBB and collection staff, including the time period between cord clamping and collection, the method of delivery and how protracted the labor time is, damage to the cord and placenta during the delivery process, and size of the placenta, all of which may impact upon the collection volume obtained and contamination of the unit. However, a robust training program for collection personnel to ensure the best possible collection in terms of aseptic process, volume obtained, and integrity of the product from the collection site to the processing laboratory is within the control of the CBB and is the foundation upon which cryopreservation of a quality product is built. With the increasing complexity of CBU donor and product qualification comes the need to recognize that the criteria change as more information is gained, such as emerging infectious diseases, new assays, and CBU use. As the technologies improve and the field of CBT transplantation evolves and matures, an active process is in place across CBBs to constantly refine and improve qualification criteria.

8.6 Future Direction

The future directions of CBU donor and product qualification are directly related to an evolving field. CBBs need to have the ability to respond and adapt quickly. For example, new emerging infectious diseases, such as the Zika virus, require the urgent need to develop guidelines for travel and potential exposure to the virus that may impact upon placental and CBU transmission, along with the development of licensed tests and mandated testing requirements. The potential serious implications of exposure to Zika virus means that as each new piece of information is discovered, new rules and procedures are set in place by CBBs, who need to respond and adapt quickly to protect the quality of banked CB.

The idea of what comprises a high-quality CBU may change over time, but SQuIPP will always be central to any assessment. The evolution and adaptation of CBBs and the CBU donor and product qualification criteria to external influences, along with the requirements of transplant programs, will ensure CBBs remain relevant and are manufacturing products of the highest quality.

References

CDC (2015) Hemoglobinopathies: current practices for screening, confirmation and follow-up. Centers for Disease Control and Prevention. https://www.cdc.gov/ncbddd/sicklecell/documents/nbs_hemoglobinopathy-testing_122015.pdf

FACT (2016) NetCord-FACT international standards for cord blood collection, banking, and release for administration, 6th edn. FACT, Nebraska

Hillyer CD (2007) Blood banking and transfusion medicine: basic principles & practice. Churchill Livingstone Elsevier, London

Hubel A et al (2003) Cryopreservation of cord blood after liquid storage. Cytotherapy 5(5):370–376

Kurtzberg J et al (2005) Results of the cord blood transplantation (COBLT) study unrelated donor banking program. Transfusion 45(6):842–855

Quinley ED (2013) Regulatory issues in transfusion medicine. In: Shaz BH, Hillyer CD, Roshal M, Abrams CS (eds) Transfusion medicine and hemostasis: clinical and laboratory aspects. Elsevier, Amsterdam

Solves P et al (2003) Comparison between two strategies for umbilical cord blood collection. Bone Marrow Transplant 31(4):269–273

9 Cord Blood Processing: Different Bags and Automation

Ludy Dobrila

9.1 Introduction

Cord blood (CB) banking is now practiced worldwide, and there are more than 100 operating public cord blood banks (CBBs) that actively contribute unrelated allogeneic hematopoietic progenitor cells (HPCs) for transplantation. Cord blood units (CBUs), voluntarily donated by delivering mothers, are harvested from the umbilical vein after the ligation of the umbilical cord (either while the placenta is still in utero or from the delivered placenta), processed, tested, and stored for eventual transplantation to unrelated recipients. There are over 700,000 donated CBUs stored in the international public CBB inventories and over 4 million CBUs stored in family CBBs for use by members of the donor's family. In this chapter, we will review the required and clinically desirable features at the end of CBU manufacturing and the diverse solutions available for the preparation and maintenance of clinically appropriate, high-quality units with long shelf lives.

9.2 Historical and Regulatory Perspective

The initial evidence of the presence of HPC in the umbilical cord blood (CB) at birth was the demonstration of hematopoietic colonies after culture of cord blood leukocytes in appropriately supplemented media reported by Knudtzon in 1974 (Knudtzon 1974). An earlier report by Ende and Ende (1972) implicated hematopoietic engraftment as the cause of blood group chimerism after the transfusion of cord blood to a young patient being treated for acute leukemia as cord blood had

L. Dobrila, Ph.D.
National Cord Blood Program, New York Blood Center, New York, NY, USA
e-mail: ldobrila@nybc.org

J. Schwartz, B.H. Shaz (eds.), *Best Practices in Processing and Storage for Hematopoietic Cell Transplantation*, Advances and Controversies in Hematopoietic Transplantation and Cell Therapy,
https://doi.org/10.1007/978-3-319-58949-7_9

been used in transfusion practice for many years (Halbrecht 1939). In 1982, Nakahata and Ogawa (1982) demonstrated the "stemness" of some cells in such colonies by obtaining tri-lineal progeny from single cell cultures. Koike and colleagues showed that frozen-stored-thawed colony-forming cells retain their hematopoietic functionality (Koike 1983). Other studies confirmed this early work and expanded on it, until, in 1988, Gluckman and colleagues performed the first human CB transplant for a patient with Fanconi anemia (FA), from an HLA-identical sibling (Gluckman et al. 1989). That successful graft has supported the recipient's blood-forming and immune functions for almost 30 years and, thus, formally established CB's ability to achieve full hematopoietic reconstitution of a bone marrow-ablated recipient. Since then, the field diversified into a family banking, where donor CBUs are reserved for use by the donor and its family, and a public banking, where donation is made voluntarily for anyone in the world who may need it.

The first public CBB (the Placental Blood Program, now, the National Cord Blood Program [NCBP]) was established at the New York Blood Center (NYBC) in 1992 by Rubinstein and colleagues (Rubinstein 1993; Rubinstein et al. 1993). They provided CBUs for the first two unrelated CB transplants in 1993 (Rubinstein et al. 1994; Kurtzberg et al. 1994). Additional public CBBs were formed rapidly in the USA, Europe, Japan, and Australia, and the numbers of CBUs stored and ready for distribution increased. The need to standardize the quality of the CBUs for transplantation leads to the first FDA Investigational New Drug (IND) approval, to the NYBC in 1996, followed by the founding of NETCORD (an international association of collaborating CBBs) in 1997 and by the involvement of FACT, an international accrediting organization in the field of clinical hematopoietic cell transplantation. The combined efforts of NETCORD and FACT led to the establishment of a joint set of FACT-NETCORD standards and to the participation of CBBs in a voluntary FACT-NETCORD accreditation program, with the first CBB accreditation awarded in 2003. The AABB, another accrediting association, subsequently established a similar program. The US FDA formally announced its intention to require the licensing of the CBUs in 2007, and the first such license was granted to NCBP in 2011. As of December 2016, seven CBBs in the USA have obtained licenses for their CBUs. Non-licensed CBUs can only be used for human transplantation under an IND approval. Thus, the CB field is formally regulated.

9.3 Rationale for an Ethnically Diverse Inventory of Frozen Publically Available Cord Blood Units

The a priori probability of finding human leukocyte antigen (HLA)-matched unrelated individuals in most human populations, particularly those including people of diverse ethnic backgrounds, is low. Hence, successful unrelated donor CB transplantation requires large numbers of cryopreserved HLA-typed CBUs to enable reasonable chances of appropriate HLA matching. Because HLA-matching requirements may be somewhat less stringent with CBU than with adult donor HPC sources (bone marrow and peripheral blood grafts), partly HLA-matched CBU can be used for transplantation. Thus, smaller numbers of donors may ensure an adequate HLA diversity. While having to freeze cells creates complications, it allows CBUs as a source of HPC an important advantage over other allogeneic HPC donor sources because of CBUs predictable availability when needed.

9.4 Cord Blood Processing

CB processing consists of preparing CBUs for freezing, which includes volume reduction and cryopreservation. Subsequently, CB is frozen, to liquid nitrogen temperature, in a rate-controlled manner (see Chap. 7). The procedure includes the preparation of aliquots to serve as testing and reference samples.

CBUs for clinical transplantation are collected into a disposable blood collection set (usually one approved for the collection of blood for transfusion), containing a citrate-based anticoagulant, usually a phosphate-buffered one (e.g., CPDA). The volume of anticoagulant relative to whole blood is important: with blood for transfusion, one volume of buffered citrate is well mixed with 7–8 volumes of fresh blood. The volume of anticoagulant is also important for CB, as the collected volume cannot be anticipated, and thus, to avoid potential clotting in the container, the anticoagulant must not be less than necessary for the collection of larger blood volumes. Since the volume of CB collected rarely exceeds 200 mL, kits containing 35 mL of anticoagulant intended for the collection of 250 mL of blood for transfusion are widely used. As a consequence, the CBU becomes larger and the CB more diluted, necessitating a larger processing container particularly after addition of facilitating agents (e.g., hydroxyethyl starch [HES]) (see Chap. 6). The volume is reduced during buffy-coat preparation. The final CBU volume should be smaller and fixed, for the following reasons: (**a**) smaller CBUs of equal, specified, size allow for organized, identified locations within a liquid nitrogen freezer facilitating individualized loading and retrieval operation; (**b**) a consistent size allows for the use of the same amount of cryopreservative (DMSO) per unit, for controlled freezing with a single cooling speed algorithm and for convenient automation of freezing; (**c**) a smaller DMSO volume, to limit DMSO infusion, particularly to pediatric recipients, as it may cause adverse events including metabolic and hemodynamic stress (see Chaps. 6 and 7).

9.4.1 Techniques for the Preparation and Extraction of Cord Blood Buffy Coats

Manually controlled or automated centrifugation can be used to separate as many of the CB leukocytes as possible into a "buffy coat," to create CBU that is preferably small, fixed, and of predetermined volume with lower hematocrit. The buffy coat contains the hematopoietic precursors ($CD34^{+}$ and hematopoietic colony-forming cells [CFCs]). However, the centrifugal separation of leukocytes from erythrocytes is not as reliably predictable as it is with the adult blood. Centrifugation losses of nucleated white cells during buffy-coat preparation are usually in the 20–40%. The lost leukocytes are trapped in the packed red cell mass. The losses may be decreased by reducing the erythrocytic ζ-(Zeta-) potential (and hence, reducing the distance between packed red cells). This has been achieved by using polymeric HES, which lowers the dielectric constant of the cell suspension and causes erythrocytes to pack more tightly, and removing the trapped leukocytes (Rubinstein et al. 1995). This facilitates the upward migration of the leukocytes originally in the lower part of the blood bag under centrifugation, through the settling red cells, and allows them to form a more complete buffy coat. While decreased with HES, the proportion of lost leukocytes remains a significant and incompletely understood individual variable when creating CB buffy coats.

1. *Manual technique*: NCBP CBU collections for research and testing purposes (not to be transfused to patients) and those made in the first 2 years of our clinical program, were collected in citrate phosphate dextrose adenine (CPDA) anticoagulant, and frozen as whole blood without volume reduction (Rubinstein et al. 1994). An equal volume of DMSO cryopreservative (20% in saline) was added slowly, with gentle and continuous mixing to the whole blood volume to reach a final DMSO concentration of 10%. The cryopreserved unit was then placed in a controlled-rate freezer. A similar method had been used to prepare the graft for the first, sibling donor CB transplant by Gluckman and colleagues (1989).

   Although the first manual CBB processing technique was efficacious (the first several dozen NCBP transplants with CBUs prepared using that procedure engrafted successfully), freezing large volumes was disadvantageous. Thus, a centrifugal volume reduction step was introduced. NCBP's early work showed that after a hard spin to make a buffy coat, a variable fraction of leukocytes stayed within the sedimented red cell bulk and was not recovered. Thus, attempting to minimize the loss, HES was added to 1% (final concentration) prior to cryopreservation and freezing. The CBU's red cells were then sedimented by soft spin centrifugation. The supernatant, including the buffy-coat layer, was transferred carefully, using a pressuring plasma extractor device, into an integral transfer bag. The leukocytes, contaminating erythrocytes and platelets in the transferred buffy-coat and plasma supernatant, were then sedimented by a second centrifugation. The excess of supernatant plasma was separated into another transfer bag, carefully avoiding resuspension of the leukocyte-containing sediment. This left a small volume of plasma and produced a leukocyte-rich cell suspension with relatively normal (40–55%) hematocrit, which was placed into a rigid 20 mL measuring jig. Then it was transferred to a freezing bag, cryopreserved with slow addition of 5 mL of 50% DMSO (in dextran 40) with continuous mixing to a final 10% concentration, before undergoing controlled-rate freezing. The resulting white blood cell (WBC) recoveries averaged 91%, and the HPC recoveries averaged 98% (Rubinstein et al. 1995). Similarly, good total nucleated cell (TNC) recoveries, i.e., TNC 87.4% and $CD34^+$ cells 90.3%, were reported by others (M-Reboredo et al. 2000).

This laborious procedure was replaced by a second, simpler, but still manual process in 1997, when Pall Medical introduced an NYBC-designed freezing bag set that enabled the storage of the cryopreserved buffy coat in a special freezing bag with two compartments (with 80% and 20% of the total capacity of 25 mL). The 20% content of the small compartment could be used for stem/progenitor cell expansion, while the contents of the larger compartment would remain frozen during the expansion culture, thus ensuring the presence of unexpanded stem cells. This bag set system has been adopted by manufacturers of automated equipment (see text below), and a large part of the currently available CBU inventory is frozen in "20–80" bags containing 5 and 20 mL, respectively. The integral plastic tubing that allowed closed-system transfer of the unit after cryopreservation was designed to allow the formation of several "segments" to contain samples of the CBU that would represent exactly the unit's content and its exposure history.

2. *Leukocyte filtration and recovery method*: Reversible leukocyte adhesion on blood filters has been proposed, developed, and tested as a method to easily trap and recover hematopoietic progenitors, by reverse flushing with a protein-enriched saline solution or other reagents (Dal Cortivo et al. 2000; Yasutake et al. 2001; Tokushima et al. 2001; Eichler et al. 2003; Shima et al. 2013).

   One comparison study (Takahashi et al. 2006) evaluated two filter systems for processing CB (developed by Asahi Kasei Medical and Terumo, respectively) versus both the manual HES method with two centrifugation steps (similar to the second manual technique, described above) and the top and bottom (T&B) method, followed by a single centrifugation (technique #4 below). This study showed that both filtration methods' median TNC recoveries were lower (58% and 61%) compared to the TNC recoveries using the traditional centrifugation methods (HES 79% and T&B 86%). MNC recovery was highest with T&B method (91%) and reduced with filters (77% and 70%) and HES method (72%). However, the $CD34^+$ cell recovery was comparable with the four methods. The selective loss of live granulocytes is likely due to their filter adherence resulting in activation with eventual apoptosis.

   A more recent report (Sato et al. 2015) evaluated the CellEffic CB (Kaneka Corporation), a novel filter for CB processing, in comparison to the Sepax system (technique 5a below). No statistically significant differences were encountered between the results of these two methods with regard to $CD45^+$ (76.1% vs. 76.6%), MNC (79.3% vs. 79.8%), and $CD45^+/CD34^+$ cell recoveries (75.2% vs. 68.6%).

3. *Improved manual method*: A manual platform based on a different principle is PrepaCyte®-CB Cord Blood Processing System (BioE, Inc., St. Paul, MN), which is FDA 510(k)-cleared. PrepaCyte®-CB is a sterile device composed of three integrally attached processing and storage bags; the first bag contains the proprietary PrepaCyte-CB separation solution. This proprietary reagent is designed to facilitate rapid agglutination and sedimentation of red blood cells. After sedimentation, the TNC-rich supernatant is expressed into the second bag for centrifugation and centrifuged without separating the bags. After this

centrifugation step, the unwanted second supernatant is returned to the first bag, maintaining "closed" status. The TNC pellet in the second bag is suspended again in a small volume, DMSO is added for cryopreservation, and the total content transferred to the third "freezing" bag for controlled-rate freezing. BioE may offer modifications of the separation solutions and other bag configurations. The system's interconnected, closed-bag set accelerates manipulations and may improve recoveries. There are few reports analyzing the effectiveness of this procedure, and in the most detailed one (Basford et al. 2010), its performance results were similar to that of Sepax ($CD45^+$ cell recoveries were 75.79% with Sepax and 72.03% with PrepaCyte). With the PrepaCyte method, recoveries of nucleated cells and $CD34^+$ cells were independent of CBU volume, whereas with the other methods discussed (hetastarch, Sepax, and plasma depletion), the recoveries decreased as the volume of CB increased (Basford et al. 2010). Regan et al. reported good results in nine patients transplanted with PrepaCyte-CB (Regan et al. 2011).

4. *Semiautomated methods*: The top and bottom method takes advantage of devices like the Optipress II Automated Blood Component Extractor (Baxter Healthcare Corp.) or the Compomat G4 (Fresenius). These instruments, developed for blood banking to enable separating donated blood units into three fractions (packed red cells, platelets, and plasma), have been also used to harvest buffy coats. The instruments may be configured to allow the separation of a buffy-coat fraction instead of platelets. Some, but not all, investigators report very good average recoveries of TNC, $CD34^+$ cells, and CFU ((Ademokun et al. 1997), TNC 90%, total progenitors 88%, $CD34^+$ cells 100%, final volume of 44 mL; (Armitage and colleagues 1999), TNC 92%, MNC 98%, $CD34^+$ cells 96%, CFU 106%, final volume 25 mL; (Takahashi and colleagues 2006), TNC 86%, MNC 91%, $CD34^+$ cells 96%; (Lapierre and colleagues 2007), TNC 61%, CD34+ cells 82%, final volume 21 mL). However, there are few recent reports on cell recovery in the context of routine CB banking for the clinical transplantation requirements. Recently, Macopharma has introduced the MacoPress Smart EVO instrument, which seems similar, though more automated. One article of its use in CB processing (Ivolgin and Smolyaninov 2014) also reported comparable TNC recoveries using the MacoPress Smart (82%) with those using Sepax (82%) and better than with manual double centrifugation (73%) (Ivolgin and Smolyaninov 2014).
5. *Automated methods*:
   (a) Sepax (Biosafe, Eysins, Switzerland), FDA 510K approved, introduced in 2000, is now used by many CBBs. It automatically separates CB leukocytes from red cells and plasma. The Sepax system (Fig. 9.1) consists of a centrifugal device (which includes a pneumatic circuit, a valve system, a microcomputer, and a LCD display) and a single-use kit (includes a harness kit and a separation chamber with a transfer piston) (Fig. 9.2). Its core device works by making the unique cylindrical disposable spin around its vertical axis, so that the CB cells are pushed against its walls not against its movable bottom. The bottom is a compressed-air-movable, computer-controlled piston which moves down, from an initial position at the top of the (empty) disposable cylinder, to transfer the CBU into its chamber. This vacuum-producing movement suffices

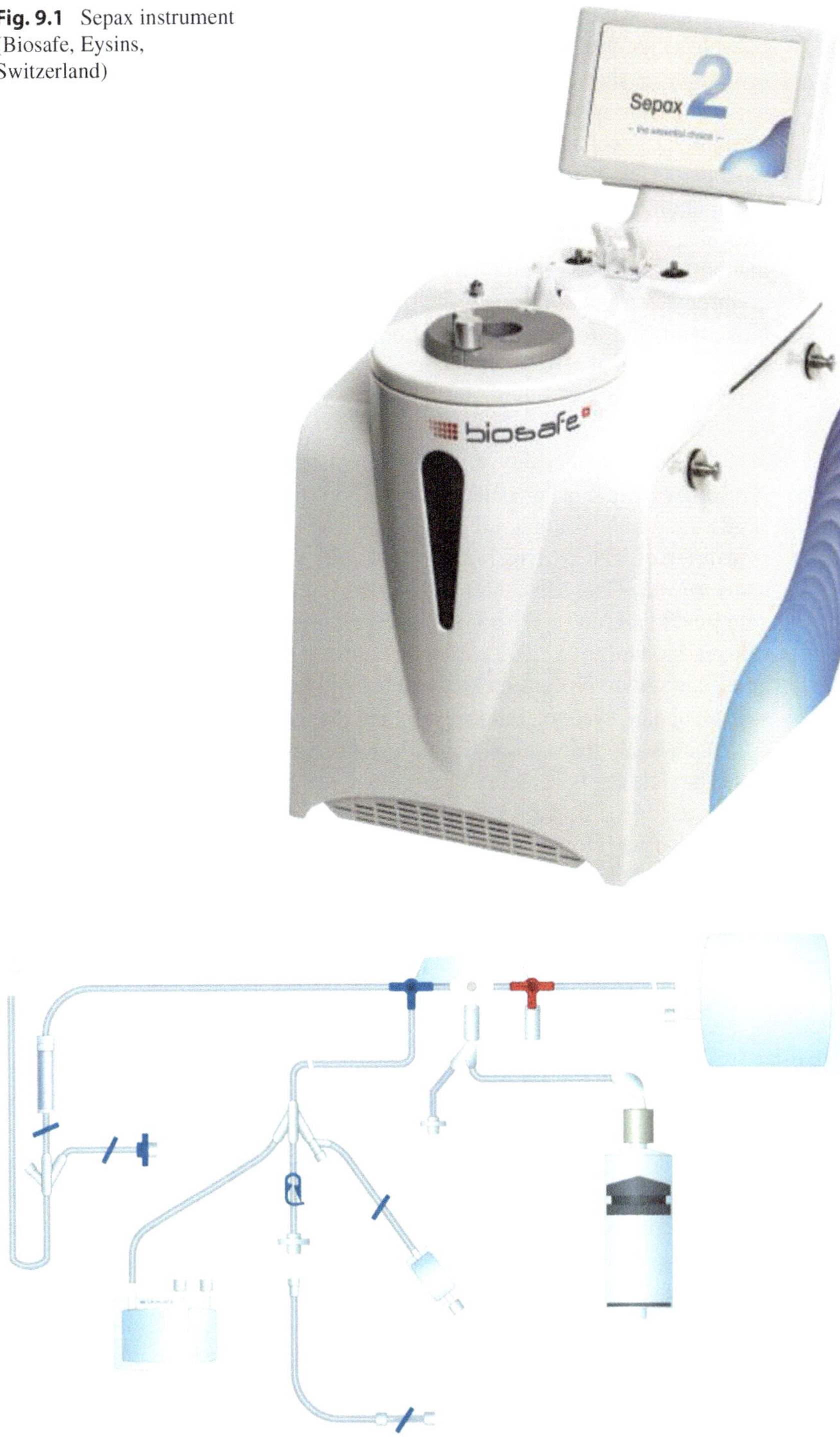

Fig. 9.1 Sepax instrument (Biosafe, Eysins, Switzerland)

Fig. 9.2 Sepax processing kit (Biosafe)

to aspirate the CB (alone or premixed with HES, usually to 1%) into the disposable's chamber. During centrifugation, the CB is separated into concentric layers: the erythrocytes further toward the circular wall, displacing the lighter leukocytes into an inner layer. After centrifugation is complete and while centrifuging at lower speed, the piston is moved upward, as the exit valve at the top opens. The plasma streams through the open valve, into sterile-docked distribution tubing leading it into an empty sterile bag. Under sensor control, the valve switches the outflowing leukocyte suspension into a different tube that connects into a second bag, which is the freezing bag. Sensing the rising erythrocytes triggers the computer to shut the valve closed, stop the piston's movement, and stop the centrifugation. The red cell bulk is left inside the disposable but can also be harvested into a third container. Average recovery after Sepax processing is reportedly TNC 76–87% and CD34$^+$ cells 86%, with 36–45% hematocrit (Lapierre et al. 2007; Rodriguez et al. 2004; Zingsem et al. 2003). TNC recovery is generally higher with CBUs of smaller volume. It also rises when using HES. According to one study (Meyer-Monard et al. 2012), the unit's volume rather than the TNC count significantly affects the recoveries of TNC, MNC, and CD34$^+$ cells with Sepax. The average TNC recovery was 77%, MNC 85%, and CD34$^+$ cells 79%, while units with initial volume <90 mL and >170 mL exhibited a similarly poor processing efficiency (Meyer-Monard et al. 2012). In order to increase the TNC recoveries in large units, a modified processing kit (double bag) was developed and used recently with an updated version of the instrument (Sepax 2) (Naing et al. 2015). Sepax 2 is functionally the same as Sepax 1, with changes to the user interface and a better module for traceability (Naing et al. 2015). With this method and without the use of HES, the final volume collected post-processing was increased to 30 mL (vs. routine volume of 20 mL) and the average TNC recoveries increased by 14% (from 75% to 89%) (Naing et al. 2015) as did the CD34$^+$ cells yield, although the hematocrit increased as well (Naing et al. 2015). Costs tend to be higher than with other automated devices. A helpful device by Biosafe, the "Coolmix," enables the timed injection of DMSO into the CBU while efficiently mixing and maintaining the set temperature of the blood until the cryopreservative addition is finished.

(b) AutoXpress® (AXP) system, Cesca Therapeutics (formerly Thermogenesis Corp.), FDA 510K approved, introduced in 2005, is the other fully automated system. The AXP system consists of (1) a hard plastic, battery-powered, microprocessor-controlled AXP device (Fig. 9.3), designed to fit in the standard carrier cups of regular blood bank centrifuges; (2) a disposable bag set, comprising three connected bags (for closed processing) (Fig. 9.4); (3) a charging station (docking station); and (4) a computer software package, XpressTRAK. An integral circuit board in the device operates a stopcock valve, part of the disposable. For the volume reduction, the CB is transferred from the collection bag, through sterile-docked tubing into the disposable's main bag, just before centrifugation. AXP may process CB with or without HES. However, the addition of HES could result in the total

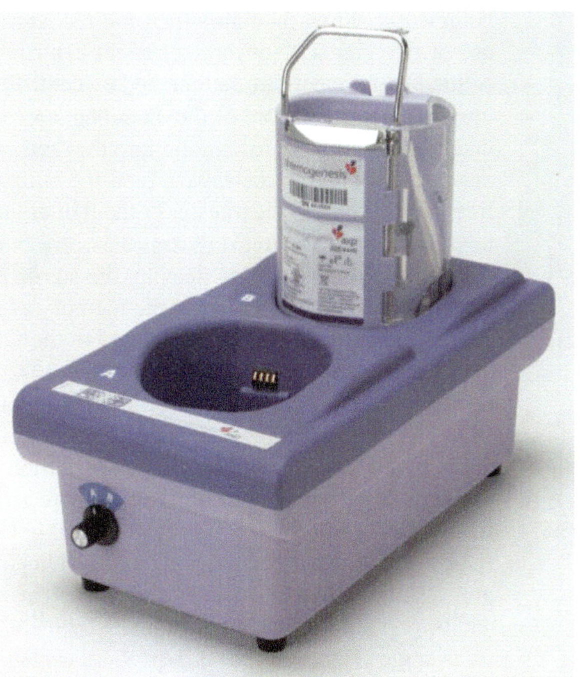

Fig. 9.3 AXP device in docking station (Cesca)

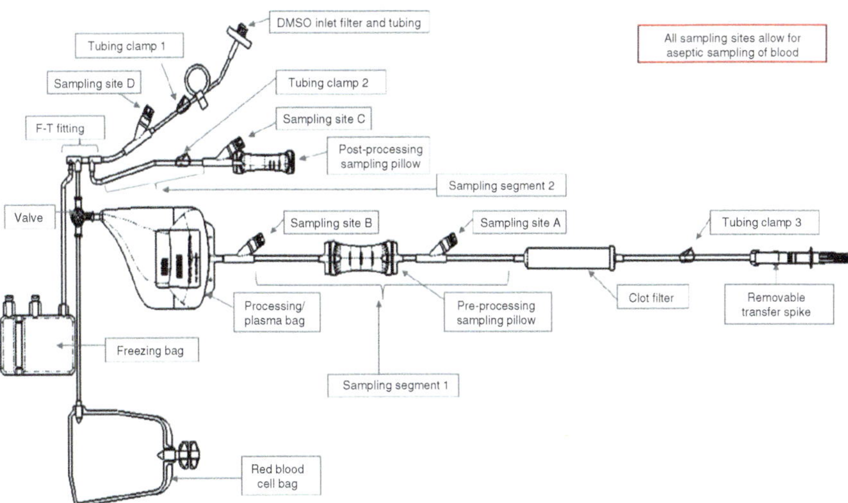

Fig. 9.4 AXP processing bag set (Cesca)

volume exceeding the limits for good recoveries and, thus, may require the use of two bag sets for more efficient centrifugal separation. After the CB cellular components are sedimented by centrifugation, the AXP valve opens the tubing at the bottom of the main bag, and the erythrocyte bulk transfers under low- speed centrifugation into the "red cell bag." As the red cell concentration decreases, the valve directs the buffy coat to the inlet tubing of the freezing bag. When the transfer of the lighter buffy-coat fraction reaches the target weight in the freezing bag, the valve closes; the CB product will be ready for cryopreservation, leaving the sterile plasma in the main bag. The performance data are stored in the memory of the AXP device's microprocessor and automatically downloaded to the CBB's laboratory information management system (LIMS), while the device's batteries recharge in the docking station. The AXP system uses the tubing of the bag set to provide in-line "sampling pillows" for separating sterile pre- and post-centrifugation test samples under closed processing conditions.

The AXP system used without HES recovers >95% MNC and >98% $CD34^+$ cells and averages 76–85% of the TNC with high viabilities >95% (Dobrila et al. 2006; Solves et al. 2013). Hematocrit is below 30%, and post-processing volume is constant and consistent with the target volume. HES addition to the AXP method significantly increases TNC recoveries by 20% on average (Dobrila et al. 2014). Similar results were obtained with large units (volume >170 mL) in which MNC recoveries improved with the addition of HES to the AXP method (MNC recoveries 99%) (Li et al. 2007).

(c) A new fully automated CB processing system, the SynGenX-1000™ (SynGen, Inc.), FDA 510K approved, is now available. The SynGenX-1000's disposable cartridge is made of hard polycarbonate, has internal sections accessed through separate tubing for red cells and buffy coat, and has a main section for the incoming blood. Loading the CBU is done through sterile-docking the collection bag's integral tubing to the disposable's sterile tubing inlet. The loaded disposable is operated by a programmable microprocessor-driven control module that fits under the disposable cartridge (Fig. 9.5) inside the standard 750 mL carrier of standard blood bank centrifuges. The battery-driven microprocessor is guided by four optical sensors that monitor the optical densities at strategic sites during the centrifugation and control the consecutive, separate transfer of the red cell and buffy-coat fractions to their respective compartments within the disposable. The plasma is left in the main section. Experience is still limited, but this device's microprocessor system provides much flexibility in the design of operation schemes and functional algorithms. The special bag set (Fig. 9.6), "CryoPRO-2," includes a DMSO-mixing chamber, the freezing bag, and sampling "bulb." An accessory, the CryoPRO Workstation, controls and documents the temperature, flow rate, and mixing of cryopreservative solutions with the buffy-coat fraction. It generates reports through dedicated "DataTRAK" software, facilitating cGMP best practices compliance. Reported results of CB processing are limited, but cell recoveries are in the same range observed with other fully automated systems. Kumar and

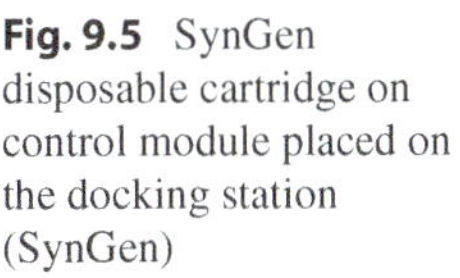

Fig. 9.5 SynGen disposable cartridge on control module placed on the docking station (SynGen)

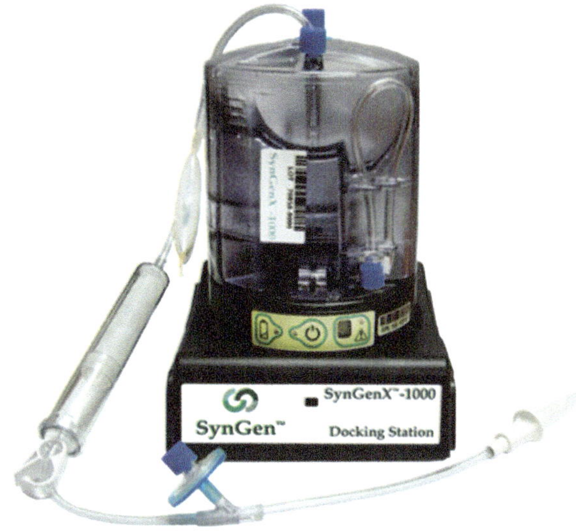

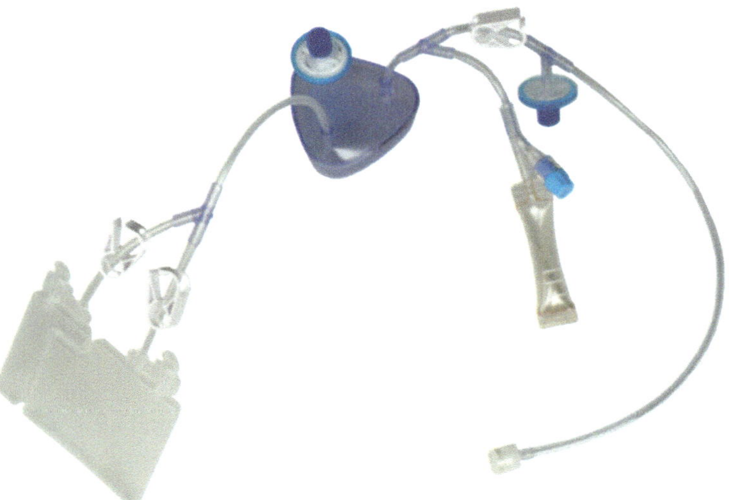

Fig. 9.6 SynGen CryoPRO-2 cryopreservation/storage bag set (SynGen)

colleagues (Kumar et al. 2014) reported recoveries of TNC 87%, MNC 94%, and CD34+ cell 102%. More recently, the Anthony Nolan Cell Therapy Centre (Lowe and Fickling 2015) showed a 12% increase in the TNC recovery when SynGen device was compared to Sepax (86% TNC recovery with SynGen vs. 74% with Sepax) and similar results for the MNC recovery (98% MNC recovery with SynGen vs. 89% with Sepax). SynGen's programming flexibility and mechanical flow characteristics allow for procedural changes as additional information is gathered in the future.

9.5 Expert Point of View

CB processing for clinical transplantation is now widely practiced under an FDA's regulatory framework that provides substantial guidance and control to CBBs.

Currently, CB banking requires FDA licensure, and CBUs can only be administered to patients in the USA if they are either FDA licensed or under FDA IND, i.e., within a clinical trial. Licensed CBUs have a regulated and validated process, including the donor variables, the containers, the means of transportation, the timing and temperature during transport, the time between birth and completion of freezing, the environmental controls needed, the conditions for CBUs while being transported and processed and under long-term storage after cryopreservation and freezing, the infectious disease testing, etc. An important requirement is demonstration of stability during the shelf life of CBUs. Licensure requires full compliance with all prerequisites, while some CBUs, which do not formally comply with all of them, may qualify as investigational units that can be transplanted under an FDA IND. CBBs may also need accreditation from either FACT or AABB. The accreditation process allows for a collegial exploration of processing techniques and their actual performance under routine conditions, within an incisive inspection of all aspects of the CBB's performance and documentation. Thus, regulated CB use in transplantation is safe and well controlled.

There are, however, challenges to CB manufacturing that must be overcome and opportunities to do so, with automated technologies becoming increasingly useful. Manual procedures are labor-intensive and error-prone, as manufacturing performance becomes increasingly detailed and complex, and computerized tools and information technology (including a laboratory information system) become more useful and effective. Automation and IT controls can be helpful in ensuring accuracy, reproducibility, and overall reliability in operations and documentation.

The difficulty of quantitatively retrieving most leukocytes from CBUs, as compared with adult donor blood, has still not been fully answered. This phenomenon has been attributed to lower deformability of a large fraction of neonatal erythrocytes, which would prevent their ability to concentrate tightly on centrifugation and push out the lighter leukocytes. In addition to erythrocyte lower membrane deformability and loss of membrane surface, close packing of the settling erythrocytes is diminished by the low plasmatic macroglobulin concentration which results in a raised dielectric constant. HES remains the most frequently used method to enhance the TNC recoveries. However, the effectiveness of adding HES is variable. Helpful innovations in methods for centrifugal separation of the buffy coat have thus far not been able to fully circumvent this problem, and further study on its mechanisms is required. Leukocyte losses are important, as the proportion of CBUs with originally high TNC counts (the index of quality most used by clinicians (Rubinstein 2009)) is relatively low, especially in African-American and some Asian neonates (probably the ethnic groups most in need for CBU for transplantation).

Lately, there has been unease among neonatologists and pediatricians regarding the time allowed for the placental transfusion, prior to ligating the umbilical cord.

Longer times before clamping the cord reduce the amount of blood left in the placental and umbilical cord veins and the eventually recoverable CB volume. The idea is to prevent iron deficiency and its manifestations in the donor infant, an important consideration especially in locales where donor infants' nutrition may not adequately maintain the donors' iron stores. Hence, the importance of improving the ability to recover leukocytes into the buffy coat is rising as higher CBU TNC numbers are associated with increased potency in transplantation, although the recovery of monocytes and $CD34^+$ cells is already quite good. No recent studies have been reported on the cell types most associated with the speed and quality of CBU transplant engraftment.

9.6 Future Directions

In addition to its critical role in determining the clinical suitability for HPC transplantation of frozen CBUs, the performance of the processing component is an important factor of cost/revenue balance in CB banking. This is largely due to the TNC losses. These losses cause a lower proportion of collected CBUs that meet the threshold criterion for TNC content, as well as to a higher proportion of over-the-threshold CBUs with relatively less competitive TNC content in the CBU inventory. Thus, improved understanding of the causes of TNC loss is critical for both clinical and financial reasons. CB high costs are due to the disproportion between the number of units added to the CBU inventory and the number of CBUs transplanted, which has remained stable or decreased in the past few years. The efficacy of the expensive methods for expanding the numbers of $CD34^+$ cell in CB grafts through pretransplantation culture with Notch ligand (Delaney et al. 2010) or through co-culturing with mesenchymal-stromal cells (MSCs) (de Lima et al. 2012) or after in vitro culture with a copper chelator (with or without nicotinamide (Horwitz et al. 2014)) has been demonstrated, as has the effectiveness of in vitro treatments of CBUs with fucosyltransferase (Popat et al. 2015). There is, however, little clinical experience, and it is not clear now whether these techniques will have a broad impact on public CB banking.

Thus, CB processing's role must also include improving the usefulness of CB banking for purposes other than HPC transplantation. Some examples of such improvement, the uses of CB plasma, for ophthalmic treatments include Sjogren's disease and acute graft-versus-host disease (aG*v*HD) (Versura et al. 2013), and of platelet lysate as a culture medium for laboratory and clinical cell expansion (Parazzi et al. 2010; Bieback 2013; Astori et al. 2016).

CB processing also needs to anticipate future requirements of clinical practice. Thus, during the 1990s, we understood the potential need for expansion of hematopoietic progenitors and worked with Pall to introduce the two-compartment freezing bags now in routine use (Rubinstein 2009). Similarly, reference samples stored with the CBU are now required for the evaluation of the stability and quality of such CBUs, which required the adoption of the "segment" samples enabled by the tubing of the CB freezing bags.

New reference samples may be required, e.g., (1) for regenerative medicine, where assays of genetic balance and stability of the CD34$^+$ and possibly mesenchymal stem and other cells may become necessary, and (2) for the determination of the suitability of a CB's immune cells for clinical use as regulatory or effector cells.

Processing specialists must be aware of the importance of CB unique assembly of cellular resources for research and clinical application and participate actively in enabling their development. Technical advances in the CB processing and regulatory requirements must be accomplished and met. Overall, however, public CB banking is a vibrant part of medical progress all over the world and is expected to supply the source material to the upcoming era of cellular therapy, already under way.

References

Ademokun JA, Chapman C, Dunn J, Lander D, Mair K, Proctor SJ et al (1997) Umbilical cord blood collection and separation for haematopoietic progenitor cell banking. Bone Marrow Transplant 19:1023–1028

Armitage S, Fehily D, Dickinson A, Chapman C, Navarrete C, Contreras M (1999) Cord blood banking: volume reduction of cord blood units using a semi-automated closed system. Bone Marrow Transplant 23:505–509

Astori G, Amati E, Bambi F, Bernardi M, Chieregato K, Schäfer R, Sella S, Rodeghiero F (2016) Platelet lysate as a substitute for animal serum for the ex-vivo expansion of mesenchymal stem/stromal cells: present and future. Stem Cell Res Ther 7(1):93

Basford C, Forraz N, Habibollah S, Hanger K, McGuckin C (2010) The cord blood separation league table: a comparison of the major clinical grade harvesting techniques for cord blood stem cells. Int J Stem Cells 3:32–45

Bieback K (2013) Platelet lysate as replacement for fetal bovine serum in mesenchymal stromal cell cultures. Transfus Med Hemother 40(5):326–335

Dal Cortivo L, Robert I, Mangin C, Sameshima T, Kora S, Gluckman E et al (2000) Cord blood banking: volume reduction using 'Procord' Terumo filter. J Hematother Stem Cell Res 9:885–890

Delaney C, Heimfeld S, Brashem-Stein C, Voorhies H, Manger RL, Bernstein ID (2010) Notch-mediated expansion of human cord blood progenitor cells capable of rapid myeloid reconstitution. Nat Med 16(2):232–236

Dobrila L, Shanlong J, Chapman J, Marr D, Kryston K, Rubinstein P (2006) ThermoGenesis AXP AutoXpress platform and Bioarchive system for automated cord blood banking [abstract]. Poster presented at the EBMT/ASBMT tandem meeting, 16–20 Feb 2006; Honolulu, HI

Dobrila L, Zhu T, Zamfir D, Wang T, Tarnawski MJ, Ciubotariu R et al (2014) Increasing post-processing total nucleated cell (TNC) recovery in cord blood banking: Hespan addition in cGMP environment. Blood 124:1126

Eichler H, Kern S, Beck C, Ziegler W, Kluter H (2003) Engraftment capacity of umbilical cord blood cells processed by either whole blood preparation or filtration. Stem Cells 21:208–216

Ende M, Ende N (1972) Hematopoietic transplantation by means of fetal (cord) blood: a new method. Va Med Mon 99:276–280

Gluckman E, Broxmeyer HE, Auerbach AD, Friedman H, Douglas GW, DeVergie A et al (1989) Hematopoietic reconstitution in a patient with Fanconi anemia by means of umbilical-cord blood from an HLA-identical sibling. N Engl J Med 321:1174–1178

Halbrecht J (1939) Transfusion with placental blood. Lancet I:202–204

Horwitz ME, Chao NJ, Rizzieri DA, Long GD, Sullivan KM, Gasparetto C et al (2014) Umbilical cord blood expansion with nicotinamide provides long-term multilineage engraftment. J Clin Invest 124(7):3121–3128

Ivolgin DA, Smolyaninov AB (2014) Isolation of nucleated cells fraction from umbilical cord blood—choice of method. Cell Organ Transplantol 2(1):30–33

Knudtzon S (1974) In vitro growth of granulocytic colonies from circulating cells in human cord blood. Blood 43:357–361

Koike K (1983) Cryopreservation of pluripotent and committed hematopoietic progenitor cells from human bone marrow and cord blood. Acta Paediatr Jpn 25:275–283

Kumar V, Perea J, Zhu T, Zamfir D, Dobrila L, Rubinstein P (2014) Processing and cryopreserving cord blood units using the SynGenX™-1000 Platform [abstract]. Poster presented at: the cord blood forum conference, 5–7 June 2014; San Francisco, CA

Kurtzberg J, Graham M, Casey J, Olson J, Stevens CE, Rubinstein P (1994) The use of umbilical cord blood in mismatched related and unrelated hematopoietic stem cell transplantation. Blood Cells 20:275–283

Lapierre V, Pellegrini N, Bardey I, Malugani C, Saas P, Garnache F et al (2007) Cord blood volume reduction using an automated system (Sepax) vs a semi-automated system (Optipress II) and a manual method (hydroxyethyl starch sedimentation) for routine cord blood banking: a comparative study. Cytotherapy 9:165–169

Li Z, Zhu H, Nguyen M, Emmanuel P, Baker B, Marr D, et al. (2007) Validation study of mononuclear cell recovery using the AXP AutoXpress platform [abstract]. Poster presented at: the EBMT meeting, 24–28 March 2007; Lyon, France

de Lima M, McNiece I, Robinson SN, Munsell M, Eapen M, Horowitz M et al (2012) Cord-blood engraftment with ex vivo mesenchymal-cell coculture. N Engl J Med 367(24):2305–2315

Lowe P, Fickling A (2015) An evaluation of the SynGenXTM processing and freezing system for implementation at Anthony Nolan Cell Therapy Centre [abstract]. Poster presented at the British Society for Gene and Cell Therapy annual conference, 9–11 June 2015; Glasgow, UK

Meyer-Monard S, Tichelli A, Troeger C, Arber C, Nicoloso De Faveri G, Gratwohl A et al (2012) Initial cord blood unit volume affects mononuclear cell and CD34+ cell-processing efficiency in a non-linear fashion. Cytotherapy 14:215–222

M-Reboredo N, Diaz A, Castro A, Villaescusa RG (2000) Collection, processing and cryopreservation of umbilical cord blood for unrelated transplantation. Bone Marrow Transplant 26:1263–1270

Naing MW, Gibson D, Hourd P, Gomez S, Horton RBV, Segal J et al (2015) Improving umbilical cord blood processing to increase total nucleated cell count yield and reduce cord input wastage by managing the consequences of input variation. Cytotherapy 17:58–67

Nakahata T, Ogawa M (1982) Hematopoietic colony-forming cells in umbilical cord blood with extensive capability to generate mono- and multipotential hematopoietic progenitors. J Clin Invest 80:1324–1328

Parazzi V, Lazzari L, Rebulla P (2010) Platelet gel from cord blood: a novel tool for tissue engineering. Platelets 21(7):549–554

Popat U, Mehta RS, Rezvani K, Fox P, Kondo K, Marin D et al (2015) Enforced fucosylation of cord blood hematopoietic cells accelerates neutrophil and platelet engraftment after transplantation. Blood 125(19):2885–2892

Regan D, Wofford J, Fortune K, Henderson C, Akel S (2011) Clinical evaluation of an alternative cord blood processing method [abstract]. Poster presented at the AABB meeting, 22–25 October 2011; San Diego, CA

Rodriguez L, Azqueta C, Azzalin S, Garcia J, Querol S (2004) Washing of cord blood grafts after thawing: high cell recovery using an automated and closed system. Vox Sang 87(3):165–172

Rubinstein P (1993) Placental blood-derived hematopoietic stem cells for unrelated bone marrow reconstitution. J Hematother 2:207–210

Rubinstein P (2009) Cord blood banking for clinical transplantation. Bone Marrow Transplant 44:635–642

Rubinstein P, Rosenfield RE, Adamson JW, Stevens CE (1993) Stored placental blood for unrelated bone marrow reconstitution. Blood 81:1679–1690

Rubinstein P, Taylor PE, Scaradavou A, Adamson JW, Migliaccio G, Emanuel D et al (1994) Unrelated placental blood for bone marrow reconstitution: organization of the placental blood program. Blood Cells 20:587–600

Rubinstein P, Dobrila L, Rosenfield RE, Adamson JW, Migliaccio G, Migliaccio AR et al (1995) Processing and cryopreservation of placental/umbilical cord blood for unrelated bone marrow reconstitution. Proc Natl Acad Sci U S A 92:10119–10122

Sato N, Fricke C, McGuckin C, Forraz N, Degoul O, Atzeni G et al (2015) Cord blood processing by a novel filtration system. Cell Prolif 48(6):671–681. https://doi.org/10.1111/cpr. 12217

Shima T, Forraz N, Sato N, Yamauchi T, Iwasaki H, Takenaka K et al (2013) A novel filtration method for cord blood processing using a polyester fabric filter. Int J Lab Hematol 35:436–446

Solves P, Planelles D, Mirabet V, Blanquer A, Carbonell-Uberos F (2013) Qualitative and quantitative cell recovery in umbilical cord blood processed by two automated devices in routine cord blood banking: a comparative study. Blood Transfus 11:405–411

Takahashi TA, Rebulla P, Armitage S, van Beckhoven J, Eichler H, Kekomäki R et al (2006) Multilaboratory evaluation of procedures for reducing the volume of cord blood: influence on cell recoveries. Cytotherapy 8(3):254–264

Tokushima Y, Sasayama N, Takahashi TA (2001) Repopulating activities of human cord blood cells separated by a stem cell collection filter in NOD/SCID mice: a comparative study of filtration method and HES method. Transfusion 41:1014–1019

Versura P, Profazio V, Buzzi M, Stancari A, Arpinati M, Malavolta N et al (2013) Efficacy of standardized and quality-controlled cord blood serum eye drop therapy in the healing of severe corneal epithelial damage in dry eye. Cornea 32(4):412–418

Yasutake M, Sumita M, Terashima S, Tokushima Y, Nitadori Y, Takahashi TA (2001) Stem cell collection filter system for human placental/umbilical cord blood processing. Vox Sang 80:101–105

Zingsem J, Strasser E, Weisbach V, Zimmermann R, Ringwald J, Goecke T et al (2003) Cord blood processing with an automated and functionally closed system. Transfusion 43:806–813

Cord Blood Graft Assessment and Selection Criteria for Transplantation

10

Andromachi Scaradavou

10.1 Introduction

Cord blood (CB) grafts extend the availability of allogeneic hematopoietic cell transplant (allo-HCT) for patients who do not have suitable adult donors, particularly those of ethnic minorities (Barker et al. 2010a; Scaradavou et al. 2013). Critical in the success of the overall transplantation is the selection of the best cord blood unit (CBU) as the graft.

Based on knowledge of CB banking and testing standards as well as experience with CB searches, this chapter aims to address aspects of CBU assessment and how these can be used for CB graft selection for transplant, including assays to evaluate the quality/potency of the CBU, interactions between TNC dose and HLA mismatch, selection of CBU with "permissible" HLA mismatches, and other graft characteristics that need to be considered.

This information pertains to CBU to be used as single or double-unit grafts for hematopoietic reconstitution of unrelated recipients with hematologic and non-hematologic diseases but does not apply fully to other uses of CB, as in regenerative medicine or adoptive cell therapies.

A. Scaradavou, M.D.
National Cord Blood Program, New York Blood Center, New York, NY, USA

Bone Marrow Transplant Service, Department of Pediatrics, Memorial Sloan-Kettering Cancer Center, New York, NY, USA
e-mail: ascaradavou@nybc.org; scaradaa@mskcc.org

J. Schwartz, B.H. Shaz (eds.), *Best Practices in Processing and Storage for Hematopoietic Cell Transplantation*, Advances and Controversies in Hematopoietic Transplantation and Cell Therapy,
https://doi.org/10.1007/978-3-319-58949-7_10

10.2 Cord Blood Unit Quality/Potency

One important aspect of quality is the potency, which indicates the engraftment potential of a CB product. Since no assays are available for the true hematopoietic stem cells (HSCs), other cells have been used as surrogates for estimating the engraftment potential and comparing CB graft characteristics.

10.2.1 Potency Evaluation of Cord Blood Unit Before Cryopreservation

Counting the number of TNC, which includes both white blood cells and nucleated red blood cells, is technically well standardized, reproducible, and accurate. TNC correlates significantly with hematopoietic progenitors such as colony-forming units (CFU) or CD34$^+$ cells and with transplant outcome endpoints such as myeloid engraftment and transplant-related mortality (TRM). TNC dose, therefore, has been the most universally accepted measurement of potency of a CBU. However, certain limitations exist: there is considerable variability of the number of hematopoietic progenitor cells (HPCs) among CBU with similar TNC. Further, the pre-cryopreservation TNC varies depending on the method of CBU processing (removal of granulocytes or no removal of cells at all). As a result, comparison of TNC among CBU that have underdone processing with different methods (e.g., automated processing versus no red blood cell depletion) may not be accurate.

HPCs are better predictors of engraftment and survival. These are evaluated by flow cytometry or functional assays.

Evaluation of the number of CD34$^+$ cells and their viability (by 7-AAD exclusion) is routinely performed by CB banks. Although most laboratories follow ISHAGE guidelines (Keeney et al. 1998), significant variability in the results exists so that it is difficult to compare values for CBU selection.

Early single institution studies showed that time to engraftment correlated with the post-thaw CD34$^+$ cell dose of the CBU (Wagner et al. 2002; Laughlin et al. 2001). A more detailed evaluation in patients who received double-unit grafts after myeloablative conditioning chemotherapy showed very good correlation of time to neutrophil recovery with the infused viable CD34$^+$ cell dose of the engrafting CBU (Purtill et al. 2013). The findings indicate that not only the number of CD34$^+$ cells after thawing but their quality also becomes important for engraftment (Purtill et al. 2013). CD34$^+$ cell viability, measured by flow cytometry with 7-AAD exclusion, was shown to be the critical determinant of engraftment in double-unit grafts, since units with CD34$^+$ cell viability below 75% had a very low probability of engraftment (Scaradavou et al. 2010). Further, low CD34$^+$ cell viability correlated with low numbers of colony-forming cells (Scaradavou et al. 2010). These findings indicate that CD34$^+$ cell viability can be a surrogate for overall CBU quality: CBU with low percentage of viable CD34$^+$ cells have a significant proportion of the CD34$^+$ cells destroyed; the remaining cells, although "viable" (i.e., not dead as determined by 7-AAD staining), are likely damaged also. As a result, the engraftment potential of the entire CBU is compromised.

Studies evaluating colony-forming units (CFU) pre-cryopreservation (Migliaccio et al. 2000) or post-thaw (Prasad et al. 2008; Page et al. 2011) have identified this measurement as the primary correlate with engraftment. However, assays for CFU have broad interlaboratory variability. The traditional CFU assay is operator dependent and the results cannot be reproduced. To this end, significant progress has been made with the New York Blood Center (NYBC) CFU strategy, an approach that combines the traditional assay with high-resolution digital imaging and storage of the electronic images so that the colonies can be classified, enumerated, and reviewed at any later point (Albano et al. 2008, 2009). Further, standardization was achieved, and results between two testing laboratories on the same samples correlated closely (Albano et al. 2011). This approach has been used successfully for thousands of CBU prior to cryopreservation, as well as for segment potency evaluation (see text in Sect. 10.2.2) at NYBC. However, this method has not been adopted by other laboratories.

Additional approaches to overcome the technical challenges of CFU assays have only been tried in very limited numbers of samples. For example, the 7-day CFU assay (Nawrot et al. 2011) has similar technical limitations as the traditional 14-day test and provides less information, and the HALO (HemoGenix, Colorado Springs, CO) functional assay, based on intracellular ATP levels related to cellular proliferation (Reems et al. 2008), only provides an indirect assessment of HSC function with limited data so far.

In summary, despite important limitations, TNC dose remains the potency measure used during the *initial* CBU assessment from the review of a search so that some potential units can be identified and subsequently evaluated in detail. Additional potency indicators, such as $CD34^+$ cell count and viability by flow cytometry and CFU assays, need to be considered, particularly when evaluating CBU with a similar TNC.

10.2.2 Potency Assays on the Cord Blood Unit Attached Segment

Ongoing studies are evaluating use of cells from the segment, the tubing integrally attached to the cryopreservation bag (Fig. 10.1), for evaluation of $CD34^+$ cell content and viability, and CFU assays, as indicators of CBU quality post-cryopreservation (Albano et al. 2009; Scaradavou et al. 2016; Rogriguez et al. 2005). There are some considerations to the use of the frozen-thawed segment for assessment of potency: it is a delicate sample that has to be handled carefully, and the laboratory performing the assays needs to have experience with such samples and interpretation of the results. Further, the freezing conditions of segment and cryopreservation bag must be similar for the quality of the segment to be representative of that of the CBU bag. Of note, the evaluation of the segment is not standardized, and intralaboratory variability applies to those results as well.

NYBC has studied CBU segments and respective thawed CBU bags to evaluate whether the segment results are representative of the CB products (N = 45) (Scaradavou et al. 2016). The total number of viable $CD34^+$ cells of the segment

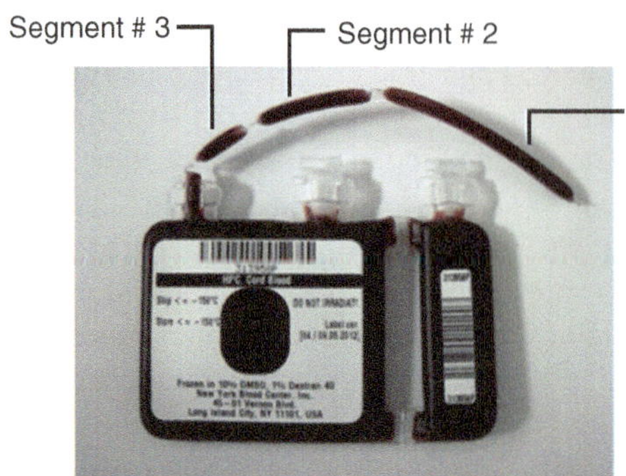

AXP CBU Attached Segments

1: HLA Confirmatory Typing

2: CD34+ cell count/viability;
CD45+ cell count/viability;
CFU testing

3: retention sample

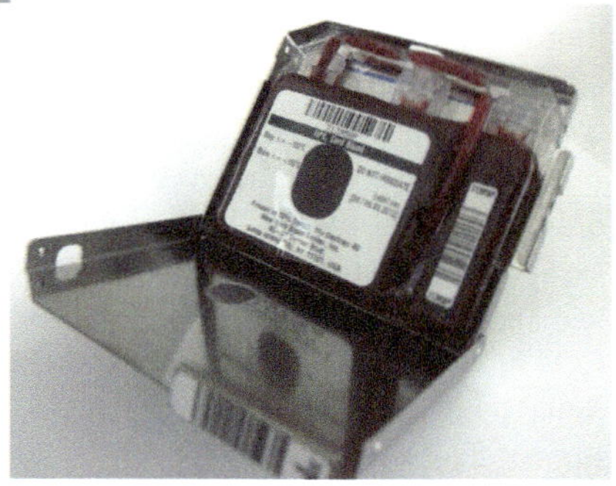

Fig. 10.1 CBU in cryopreservation bag with the attached segments; position of segments in the metal canister

correlated highly with the number of viable CD34⁺ cells obtained from the thawed bag ($r = 0.93$, $p < 0.01$). Similarly, CFU of the segment correlated well with the thawed bag CFU ($r = 0.68$, $p < 0.01$) (Scaradavou et al. 2016). Additionally, good correlation of the segment results with those obtained from the CBU after thawing has been shown for small numbers of samples by other CB banks (Rogriguez et al. 2005; Querol et al. 2010).

Further, NYBC recently presented results for a total of 1924 segments of approximately 1500 CBU processed with the AutoXpress (AXP) (Cesca Therapeutics, Rancho Cordova, CA) automated system over a period of 10 years (2006–2016); some CBU are cryopreserved in two bags, and in those cases, both segments were evaluated. All these CBU have been released for transplantation (Scaradavou et al. 2016). Flow cytometry evaluation with 7-AAD exclusion showed that mean segment $CD34^+$ viability was 96%, median was 96.5%, and standard deviation (SD) was 3.5% (median time in storage, 2.3 years). The analysis also showed that segment $CD34^+$ cell viability correlated with the CFU output of the HPCs from the segment and, therefore, indicated that the $CD34^+$ cell viability is a reliable assay for CBU potency. In contrast to CFU functional assays that require 14 days, $CD34^+$ cell viability is available on the same day and provides reliable information for the cryopreserved product.

Segment evaluation, therefore, is feasible on a large-scale basis, but the results have to be evaluated with caution. Notably, $CD34^+$ cell viability is the indicator of quality, while $CD45^+$ cell viability is usually lower since it reflects the granulocytes that are dying during the freezing-thawing procedures. Importantly, $CD45^+$ cell viability has not shown to have any effect on CBU engraftment (Scaradavou et al. 2010).

Additional studies from the Duke investigators indicate that ALDH bright ($ALDH^{br}$) cells evaluated by multiparameter flow cytometry correlated closely with CFU assay results in almost 4000 CBU segments (Shoulars et al. 2016). Segment $ALDH^{br}$ content presents a fast way to evaluate the potency of the cryopreserved CBU (Wagner 2016), and segment results correlated with those of the respective thawed bags ($n = 60$, $r = 0.88$). Further, higher expression of $ALDH^{br}$ was associated with faster neutrophil engraftment in a small number of recipients ($n = 78$ patients, $p = 0.03$) (Shoulars et al. 2016). However, it is early to know whether this measurement could be standardized among different laboratories.

CB banks have modified their practices so that more segments are available for the recently processed CBU, to allow for prerelease testing. Occasional CBU, however, may not have a segment available for potency evaluation, especially if they were cryopreserved years ago and their (only) segment was used for HLA confirmatory typing. These CBU can be used for transplantation provided they meet the other selection criteria. Evaluation of the overall performance of the CB bank may help the decision, as well as backup plans in case of unexpected results on the day of thawing.

10.2.3 Standardization of Banking Practices and Oversight

Standardization of CB banking practices is crucial for consistent high quality of the products and reliability of testing results. Accreditation agencies (NetCord/FACT—Foundation for the Accreditation of Cellular Therapy and AABBAmerican Association of Blood Banks) evaluate CB banks for compliance with their respective standards to ensure their optimal function. A recent study evaluated $CD34^+$ cell viability for a large number of CBU obtained from domestic and international CB banks that were thawed at a single transplant center and evaluated some of the banking practices that may impact the result (Purtill et al. 2013). CB bank accreditation by FACT was shown to be an independent prognostic variable. So it is desirable to obtain CBU from accredited banks to optimize transplant outcomes.

The US FDA (Food and Drug Administration) biologics license procedures for the CB banks need to be viewed in the same context (FDA Guidance for Industry 2014). The FDA regulations focus on Current Good Manufacturing Practices (cGMPs) that ensure safety, quality, identity, potency, and purity of the product (HPC, Cord Blood). They provide assurance that all steps from CBU collection to CBU release for transplant have undergone close monitoring and review and the results meet predetermined standards. NYBC was the first CB bank to be licensed in 2011. As of September 2017, 7 US public CB banks have been licensed by the FDA, and others are in the process. CBU that are not licensed have to be used under an Investigational New Drug (IND) clinical study. Different agencies in Europe also have high standards and perform rigorous evaluations of CB banks.

10.3 Selection of Cord Blood Unit for Transplant: Influence of Total Nucleated Cell Dose and HLA-Matching for Outcomes

The interaction of TNC and HLA is a very important consideration for CBU selection. CBU-recipient HLA match was initially evaluated at the low/intermediate resolution level for HLA-A and HLA-B and allele level for HLA-DRB1 and, currently, at the allele level for HLA-A, HLA-B, HLA-C, and HLA-DRB1. In all studies, higher TNC can overcome, to some extent, HLA disparities.

10.3.1 TNC and HLA Match at HLA-A, HLA-B, and HLA-DRB1

As described in early single-institution studies, the speed of myeloid engraftment correlated with the TNC dose of the CBU, i.e., the number of TNC per kilogram of the patient's body weight (Wagner et al. 2002; Laughlin et al. 2001, 2004; Rocha et al. 2000, 2004). In the original NYBC analysis of transplant outcomes, TNC dose was the most significant graft characteristic correlating with engraftment: a stepwise improvement in the time and probability of engraftment was seen with increasing TNC doses (Rubinstein et al. 1998). In the same analysis, the role of HLA match was identified as affecting time to engraftment, transplant-related events, and survival (Rubinstein et al. 1998). Eapen and colleagues (2007) compared the outcomes of 503 children with leukemia transplanted with unrelated CB grafts to those of 282 recipients of unrelated BM. Higher TRM was seen for patients who received one HLA-mismatched CBU with low TNC (defined as $<3 \times 10^7$/kg of recipient body weight) or two HLA-mismatched CB grafts independently of cell dose. In contrast, six of six HLA-matched and five of six HLA-matched CBU with TNC $>3 \times 10^7$/kg of recipient body weight had outcomes similar to those of HLA-matched BM grafts. Similar analyses from Eurocord described a log-linear relationship between cell dose and probability of engraftment (Gluckman and Rocha 2009). These early studies recommended using CBU with ≤2 HLA mismatch and a TNC $>2.5–3.0 \times 10^7$cells/kg of recipient body weight, reflecting a clear emphasis on TNC for CBU selection rather than on HLA matching. Barker and colleagues (2010b) analyzed 1061 patients (children and adults, median age, 9.3 years; range, 0.1–64 years) who received single-unit grafts from the NYBC during the period 1993–2006 for leukemia or myelodysplasia after myeloablative cyto-reduction, to evaluate how to "trade" HLA mismatch and TNC dose. The results suggested a selection algorithm that gives priority to 0 HLA-mismatched units. In the absence of HLA-matched grafts, the recommendation was the selection of a 1 HLA-mismatched CBU with TNC $>2.5 \times 10^7$/kg of recipient body weight or a 2 HLA-mismatched CBU with TNC $>5.0 \times 10^7$/kg of recipient body weight. Further, CBU with TNC $<2.5 \times 10^7$/kg of recipient body weight, with either one or two HLA mismatch, need to be avoided (Barker et al. 2010b). Notably, neither TNC dose nor HLA match was associated with an effect on relapse. As a result, lower TRM was achieved with better HLA match without an increase in relapse rates. In other words, no advantage in selecting four of six HLA-matched units in order to increase the antileukemic effect of the graft was seen in this study.

10.3.2 TNC and HLA Match at Allele Level HLA-A, HLA-B, HLA-C, and HLA-DRB1

Analysis of a large cohort of single CBU recipients (N = 803 patients, 49% of them below the age of 10 years) for hematologic malignancies by Eapen and colleagues on behalf of CIBMTR showed that matching for HLA-C improved TRM (Eapen et al. 2011).

Further, Eapen and colleagues published results of a large retrospective analysis of 1568 single-unit CB recipients with hematologic malignancies treated with myeloablative regimens, and they evaluated allele level matching for HLA class I and the effects on non-relapse mortality (NRM) (Eapen et al. 2014). The population was primarily pediatric (only 29% of the patients were older than 16 years), and 7% of the patients received eight of eight HLA-allele-matched CBU. Fifty percent of the HLA typings, primarily those of transplants prior to 2005, were not available at the allele level, but they were imputated using the Haplogic III (high-resolution imputation algorithm). Mismatches of ≥3 alleles led to significantly higher NRM; however, overall survival was significantly lower *only* for grafts with five allele HLA mismatches. Importantly, increased TNC could help overcome HLA disparities, so CBU with higher TNC content had better outcomes despite HLA mismatches. Importantly, the risk of relapse was not associated with HLA matching (Eapen et al. 2014).

Altogether the data suggest that CBU must have a minimal TNC dose for engraftment (>3.0×10^7/kg of recipient body weight pre-cryopreservation for single-unit CB transplants according to the CIBMTR data), but above that "threshold" TNC dose, HLA allele level matching should be prioritized (Table 10.1).

These results modified the "landscape" of HLA matching for unrelated CB transplants. It becomes clear that high-resolution HLA typing has to be performed for patient and CBU and that allele level matching has to be *evaluated*. Further, significant increases in the TNC dose can overcome, to some extent, HLA disparities. Importantly, CBU selection has to prioritize HLA matching above a "threshold" TNC dose. Moreover, use of mismatched CBU does not decrease the risk of relapse but could increase NRM.

10.4 Selection of Cord Blood Unit with "Permissible" HLA Mismatches

Despite the size of the worldwide CB Inventory estimated at 720,000 CBU (Bone Marrow Donors Worldwide n.d.), only small numbers of patients (less than 10% in the studies described) will have a fully HLA-matched CBU. The vast majority of the CB recipients receive mismatched CB grafts. Thus, there has been interest in

Table 10.1 Cord blood unit selection guidelines

1. *"Screen" CBU by TNC dose: establish a TNC dose "threshold," below which CBU will not be evaluated.* TNC dose depends on the use of single or double CBU graft or additional HPC sources and on specific center studies
• Minimum TNC dose of 2–3 × 10^7/kg of recipient body weight for single CBU and 1.5–2.0 × 10^7/kg of recipient body weight for each CBU in a double graft
• Higher CBU TNC doses (4–5 × 10^7/kg of recipient body weight) recommended for nonmalignant diseases
2. For CBU above the "threshold" TNC dose
• Evaluate HLA match level (at six and eight alleles) **A six of six (or eight of eight) allele HLA-matched CBU would be the first choice—CBU quality has to be considered as in all other CBU**
• Avoid CBU with <3 of 8 allele level match, if possible
• If only HLA-mismatched CBU are available, consider "permissible" mismatches for patients with hematologic malignancies: evaluate maternal HLA for NIMA/IPA assignments, and give priority to CBU with NIMA match and/or shared IPA targets
• Evaluate potency assays; prioritize CBU with $CD34^+$ cell dose >1.0–1.5 × 10^5/kg of recipient body weight
• Prioritize accredited CB banks and licensed CB products **• Presence of CBU segment for confirmatory typing and potency evaluation**
• Do not limit selection based on unit-to-unit match for double CBU grafts
• Evaluate potential patient-related variables (DSA, RBC content, CBU volume)
3. Identify CBU for the graft; also identify backup graft

approaches identifying CBU with "permissible" HLA mismatches that do not adversely affect outcomes.

10.4.1 Fetal-Maternal Interactions during Pregnancy: NIMA Effects

The immunologic fetal-maternal interactions during pregnancy and the subsequent effects on the transplant recipients have been studied by our group and others.

The fetus inherits one HLA haplotype from the father (inherited paternal antigens—IPA) and one from the mother (inherited maternal antigens—IMA) (Fig. 10.2). During pregnancy, bidirectional transplacental trafficking of cells exposes the fetus to the maternal cells, expressing both the IMA and NIMA (non-inherited maternal antigens), resulting in NIMA-specific responses (van Rood and Oudshoorn 2009; Van Rood et al. 1958).

The first study to evaluate the impact of fetal exposure to NIMA on the outcome of unrelated CB transplants was by van Rood and colleagues in 2009 (van Rood et al. 2009). The hypothesis was that exposure to NIMA during fetal life would have an effect on transplant outcomes in cases where there was a NIMA match between recipient and CB donor. This was evaluated in 1121 patients with hematologic malignancies that received single CBU from the NYBC (van Rood et al. 2009).

Patients were assigned in three groups: (a) those with 0 HLA-mismatched grafts ($n = 62$, 6% of total), (b) those with HLA-mismatched and NIMA-matched grafts

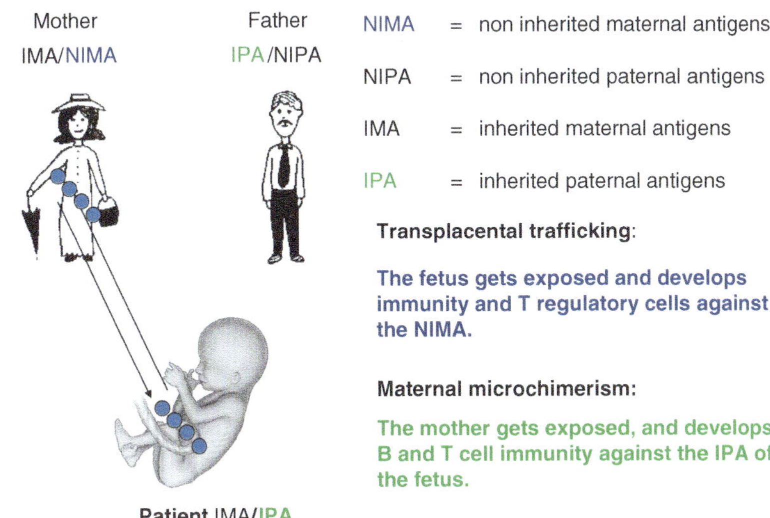

Fig. 10.2 Scheme of fetal-maternal interactions during pregnancy

(n = 79, 7% of total), and (c) those with HLA-mismatched and NIMA-mismatched grafts (n = 980). NIMA matching was assigned retrospectively; CBU were not selected based on NIMA at the time of transplant. The analysis showed statistically significant improvements in TRM for the NIMA-matched grafts compared to those of NIMA-mismatched grafts. Further, overall mortality and treatment failure for HLA-mismatched, NIMA-matched grafts were significantly improved, and engraftment was improved, particularly for patients who received lower cell dose grafts. Notably, outcomes of one HLA mismatch NIMA-matched grafts were similar to those of 0 HLA mismatch grafts. Further, posttransplant relapse tended to be lower in patients with acute myeloid leukemia (AML) that received one HLA-mismatched, NIMA-matched CB unit. There was no increased incidence of G*v*HD in recipients of HLA-mismatched, NIMA-matched CB grafts (van Rood et al. 2009).

The subsequent study by of Rocha and colleagues (Rocha et al. 2012), combining NMDP and Eurocord data, aimed to confirm the superior outcomes of HLA-mismatched, NIMA-matched CB grafts in patients with hematologic malignancies. Using a smaller patient cohort and a different type of analysis, the authors compared the results of 48 HLA-mismatched, NIMA-matched CB grafts to those of 118 patients who received HLA-mismatched, NIMA-mismatched CBU. NIMA matches were also assigned retrospectively. The frequency of NIMA-matched CB grafts was 8.5% among the 508 eligible patients. In this study also, the TRM was lower after NIMA-matched grafts; consequently overall survival (OS) was shown to be higher after NIMA-matched CB transplants. No effects on engraftment, incidence of G*v*HD, or relapse were detectable in this dataset.

In summary, these two large retrospective studies showed a beneficial role for NIMA-matched CB grafts, leading to significant improvement in posttransplant survival. Therefore, in the absence of a fully matched donor, HLA-mismatched, NIMA-matched CBU can be the graft of choice for patients with hematologic malignancies (Scaradavou 2012), and studies have addressed the positive impact of NIMA-matched CB grafts on finding donors for patients (van den Zanden et al. 2014).

10.4.2 Improved Outcomes with Cord Blood Units that Share Inherited Paternal Antigen Targets with the Recipients

Another important biological aspect of the fetal-maternal interactions is the presence of maternal microchimerism in the fetus and in the CB (Scaradavou et al. 1996). van Rood and colleagues hypothesized that the maternal cells sensitized to the fetal inherited paternal antigens (IPA), when transplanted with the CB, may have an effect on outcome when the patient has the same antigen as the IPA. In those cases, patient and CB donor "share" an IPA target for the maternal cells (van Rood et al. 2012).

A total of 845 recipients with AML or ALL that received single CBU from the NYBC was retrospectively assigned in two groups, those with CB grafts that shared IPA targets at one, two, or three HLA loci ($N = 751$) or those with no shared IPA targets ($N = 64$), representing 6% of the total patient-unit pairs (van Rood et al. 2012). The two groups were similar in regard to patient and disease characteristics and TNC doses. The incidence of acute G*v*HD grade III and IV was not different among the groups. On the contrary, there were significantly lower relapse rates in the group of HLA-mismatched but shared IPA grafts. In particular, relapse reduction was most significant in patients receiving one HLA-mismatched CB graft with shared IPA target (HR = 0.15, $p < 0.001$). The hypothesis was that the potent graft-versus-leukemia (G*v*L) effect was mediated by the maternal microchimeric cells, and it was found to be independent of other HLA associations (van Rood et al. 2012; Burlingham and Nelson 2012; Milano et al. 2013).

The above findings support avoiding CBU with no IPA targets, if possible, for patients with hematologic malignancies.

10.4.3 Direction of HLA Mismatch and Effects on Transplant Outcomes

The effect of the direction of HLA mismatch was evaluated in a study by the NYBC (Stevens et al. 2011). By definition, when a mismatched HLA is present in both recipient and donor, the mismatch is bidirectional. In contrast, if either the donor or the recipient is homozygous in one locus, the mismatch is unidirectional. Analysis of 1207 patients transplanted with single CBU from the NYBC during the period 1993–2006 revealed 98 patient-donor pairs (8.1%) that had unidirectional MM: 58 in the G*v*HD direction only (G*v*H-only mismatch) and 40 in the rejection direction only (rejection-only mismatch). Seventy patients (6% of total) had zero mismatch grafts, and this cohort was the "reference" group for the comparisons. The remaining patients had bidirectional or combination of HLA mismatch. GvH-only mismatch grafts had engraftment and TRM outcomes that were as good as those that had 0 MM and significantly better than those with one bidirectional MM. Rejection-only mismatch grafts, on the other hand, carried a higher risk of relapse and lower engraftment rate (Stevens et al. 2011).

In agreement with these results, two other CB transplant studies showed relationships between the number of mismatches in the G*v*H direction and myeloid engraftment (Ottinger et al. 2003; Matsuno et al. 2009) but did not report on G*v*HD, relapse, or survival endpoints. On the other hand, the Eurocord data analysis by Cuncha and colleagues (Cunha et al. 2014) did not support these findings. The investigators evaluated outcomes of 1565 recipients of single-unit CB grafts; of those 10% had 0 HLA-mismatched grafts. Using the five of six HLA-matched (i.e., one HLA mismatch) recipient group as "reference," no difference was seen with the unidirectional HLA mismatch. However, no association between HLA and any outcomes was seen in this study. The different population characteristics, diseases, and analytical approaches may account for the different results.

The implication of these observations is that the direction of the HLA mismatch needs to be evaluated in CBU selection so that grafts with G*v*H-only mismatch can be given priority over other types of mismatches.

10.5 Approaches to Overcome the TNC Limitations of Single CB Graft

Several novel strategies are being evaluated for their effects on CB transplant outcomes. In these treatments CBU selection depends, to some extent, on the combination of grafts and stem cell sources used.

In young pediatric patients, the CBU TNC dose is not a major obstacle: most centers aim for a pre-cryopreservation cell dose >2.5–3 × 10^7/kg of recipient body weight for patients with hematologic malignancies and >4–5 × 10^7/kg of recipient body weight for children with nonmalignant diseases, with no well-defined upper limit. The recent randomized study of one versus two CBU for pediatric patients with acute leukemia did not show advantages for double-unit grafts (Wagner et al. 2014). For larger pediatric patients, however, dose limitations exist, as is the case with most adults. In addition, even with moderate cell doses, the posttransplant neutropenia is long. In order to improve engraftment as well as decrease the period of posttransplant pancytopenia and related medical complications including prolonged hospital stay, several approaches have been investigated such as use of double-unit grafts (Barker et al. 2003, 2005; Brunstein et al. 2007, 2010; Avery et al. 2011), use of HLA-haploidentical T-cell-depleted (TCD) grafts in combination with CBU (reviewed in van Besien and Childs 2016), intrabone marrow injections, ex vivo expansion of the hematopoietic stem and progenitor cells, systemic addition of mesenchymal stem cells, and use of agents to enhance homing of CB cells to the bone marrow. These novel strategies (reviewed in Oran and Shpall 2013; Ballen et al. 2013; Ballen 2017) aim to improve the overall outcomes of unrelated CB transplantation. Their advantages and indications are outside the scope of this review; the points related to CBU selection for these different approaches are discussed briefly below.

10.5.1 Double-Unit Cord Blood Grafts

In double-unit grafts, only one CBU gives rise to long-term hematopoiesis in the majority of the cases. The time to neutrophil engraftment has been shown to correlate with the TNC dose of the engrafting CBU and, most recently, with the viable infused $CD34^+$ cell dose of the engrafting CBU (Purtill et al. 2013). Since we cannot accurately predict which unit will engraft, selection of *each* of the CBU of the graft empirically follows the criteria of single-unit grafts with a minimum TNC >1.5–2.0 × 10^7/kg of recipient body weight for five of six or four of six HLA-matched CBU and consideration of $CD34^+$ cell dose and viability (see Sect. 10.2). The role of allele level HLA matching has not been evaluated in double CBU grafts specifically, but most transplant physicians would apply the criteria of single-unit CBU selection, including evaluation at the allele level for HLA class I.

Importantly, there are no data indicating that the level of mismatch between the two units of the graft has any effect on engraftment. Avery and colleagues (2011) found no association between unit-to-unit HLA match and incidence of graft failure or speed of engraftment in 84 double CB recipients transplanted for hematologic malignancies following myeloablative cyto-reduction. Similarly, in a recent analysis of 449 patients with acute leukemia after double CB transplants, unit-to-unit HLA mismatch (<2 or 3–4 loci) had no effect in any outcome endpoints (Brunstein et al. 2017).

10.5.2 Combination Grafts

The use of another hematopoietic graft source providing hematopoietic progenitor cells, in most cases TCD, until the CB-derived cells are seen in the peripheral blood is being evaluated in several studies (see review van Besien and Childs 2016). The advantage of this approach is that CBU TNC may not be a limiting factor since the other graft is supposed to provide neutrophils during the early posttransplant period. As a result, the best HLA-matched CBU can be selected. Ongoing analyses will have to confirm if this is the case in all clinical scenarios.

10.6 Patient Diagnosis and Relapse Risk

There is no evidence to suggest a higher risk of relapse after CB transplantation. Relapse risks were not different in the comparison studies of unrelated CB or BM grafts in both pediatric (Eapen et al. 2007) and adult patients (Eapen et al. 2010), performed by CIBMTR. Further, there was no indication that HLA-mismatched grafts lead to lower posttransplant relapse rates for patients with hematologic malignancies in the NYBC analyses (Rubinstein et al. 1998) and the CIBMTR evaluations of single-unit CB grafts (Eapen et al. 2014). These studies, however, clearly showed an increase in TRM with higher HLA mismatches. As a result, there is no clinical advantage in selecting preferentially CBU with higher number of HLA mismatches for patients with hematologic malignancies. The effect of double-unit CB grafts on relapse is evaluated in retrospective (Verneris et al. 2009; Milano et al. 2016) as well as prospective studies.

Patients with nonmalignant diseases have a higher overall probability of graft failure for a variety of disease- or prior treatment-related reasons. In a recent Eurocord analysis, HLA disparity was found to have a major impact on engraftment, G*v*HD, TRM, and survival (Gluckman and Rocha 2009).

10.7 Other Immunological Considerations for Cord Blood Unit Selection

10.7.1 Donor-Specific HLA Antibodies

The impact of donor-directed specific anti-HLA antibodies (DSA) on CB engraftment has been evaluated in several studies with somewhat conflicting results. Brunstein and colleagues (2011) evaluated 126 recipients of double CB grafts and reported a comparable cumulative incidence of engraftment in DSA and non-DSA patients and no association with CB unit dominance. Moreover, Dahi and colleagues (2014a) found no effect on engraftment for patients with DSA antibodies that received double unit CB transplants after myeloablative conditioning. In contrary, Takahashi and colleagues (2010) showed significantly lower incidence of engraftment in single CB transplants after myeloablative chemotherapy for patients with CBU-specific antibodies. Similarly, Cutler and colleagues (2011) found a negative effect of DSA on engraftment of double CBU transplants in 73 patients. The incidence of graft failure was 5.5% in patients with no detectable DSA, 18.2% in the 11 patients with DSA against one of the two units, and 57% in the 9 recipients with DSA against both CBU ($p = 0.0001$). Ruggeri and colleagues (2013) reviewed the European experience of 294 patients after reduced intensity conditioning: the incidence of engraftment in the 14 patients with DSA was 44% compared to 81% for those without DSA ($p = 0.006$).

In addition to differences in patient characteristics, CBU selection, conditioning, and immunosuppression regimens, the conflicting results may also be explained by variations in HLA antibody assays and mean fluorescence intensity of the DSA. Overall, most physicians test for DSA prior to CBU selection for adult, heavily transfused patients and would avoid CBU with HLA against patients having high titer DSA.

10.7.2 KIR-Ligand Compatibility

Conflicting data exist on the effect of killer immunoglobulin receptor-ligand (KIR-L) matching in CB transplantation. The European group evaluated 218 single CBU recipients with acute leukemia (Willemze et al. 2009) and noted improved leukemia-free survival and OS in the recipients of KIR-L incompatible grafts in the GvHD direction, as well as decreased incidence of relapse. In contrast, the Minnesota group evaluated 257 recipients of single- ($n = 91$) or double-unit ($n = 166$) HLA-mismatched CB grafts after myeloablative ($n = 155$) or reduced intensity ($n = 102$) cyto-reduction and found no advantage in using KIR-L mismatched CB grafts (Brunstein et al. 2009). Subsequent studies also showed controversial results. As of now, natural killer (NK) cell-related considerations have not been incorporated into CBU selection practices, unless under specific clinical trials.

10.8 Other Graft Characteristics Affecting Cord Blood Unit Quality and Safety

10.8.1 Attached Segment: HLA Confirmatory Typing (CT)

NetCord/FACT and FDA require confirmation of the identity of the CBU by HLA typing of an attached segment prior to release for transplantation. Since mislabeling errors still can occur (McCullough et al. 2009; Murphy et al. 2016), the presence of an attached segment remains an important consideration for CBU selection for clinical use.

10.8.2 Time in Storage: "Expiration Date?"

The significance of unit "age" (i.e., length of storage time) is an area of active investigation. While there is no apparent decrease of the hematopoietic potential of CB cells that have been cryopreserved for over a decade, as evaluated by in vitro assays and mouse models (Broxmeyer et al. 2003), the importance of the collection/processing year may relate more to changing banking practices, equipment, standards, and testing assays (cryopreservation and testing for hematopoietic progenitors, infectious disease markers, and others) over time.

Several CB banks are evaluating the long-term effects of cryopreservation on the stored products. Under the FDA license, annual CBU stability studies are required. For the NYBC stability studies, clinical CBU from the different manufacturing periods are thawed, and evaluation of segment and CBU bag addresses potency, bacterial contamination, and identity of the products, as well as container and label stability. So far, CBU cryopreserved for as long as 20 years do not show a decrease in potency by in vitro assays. Based on the ongoing evaluations, the expiration date of the products that is shown on the licensed product label is being extended annually.

Further, post-thaw flow cytometric evaluation of 684 segments from "old" CBU, cryopreserved for a median of 10 years (manual processing during the period 1997–2006), showed a mean $CD34^+$ cell viability of 94.2% (median, 95.2%; SD, 4.3%)

(Scaradavou et al. 2016). These results were not different from the CD34$^+$ cell viabilities of recently cryopreserved CBU (Sect. 10.2.2).

Moreover, outcome data analysis from the NYBC showed no difference in time to engraftment, graft failure rate, and overall survival for CBU infused after cryopreservation and storage for >8 years ($n = 43$; median storage time, 9.2 years), compared to those transplanted within 2 years from collection ($n = 300$; median storage time, 1.1 years) (Scaradavou et al. 2007), indicating that long-term storage is feasible without compromising the quality and engraftment ability of the CBU. It should be noted, however, that freezing and storage procedures, equipment, and devices may vary significantly over time and from bank to bank and NYBC results may not necessarily apply to other banks.

Further, evaluation of 288 CBU from many CB banks, cryopreserved over a range of 0.8–11 years and transplanted at the University of Minnesota, showed no effect of the length of storage time to neutrophil recovery (Mitchell et al. 2015).

10.8.3 Red Cell Content of Cord Blood Unit Post-Processing

The red blood cell (RBC) content of the CBU (i.e., RBC reduced or RBC replete) may influence unit choice and CBU preparation for infusion. The RBC content can be evaluated by the post-processing hematocrit of the CBU or the total number of RBCs remaining in the product. For example, CBU processed with the AXP automated system typically have hematocrit below 50%, in most cases below 30%. In contrast, manually processed CBU have a wide range of hematocrit values, as high as 60%. Plasma-reduced but RBC-replete CBU can have hematocrits as high as 70% and usually have higher cryopreservation volumes also, so the total RBC content of the product is substantial. Although data on direct comparison of RBC-reduced and RBC-replete units may be difficult to obtain, analysis of engraftment of RBC-replete but plasma-reduced units has shown similar results to the partially RBC-depleted grafts (Chow et al. 2007; Nikiforow et al. 2017). However, important concerns remain about the significant load of RBC debris and free hemoglobin of these units upon thawing (Barker and Scaradavou 2011) and the serious, sometimes fatal, infusion adverse events that have been reported (NMDP n.d.), if the products are not washed prior to infusion. Current recommendations require washing of RBC-replete CBU prior to infusion and hydration and careful monitoring of the patients. On the other hand, washing post-thaw may result in high WBC losses due to the difficulty of separating the supernatant from the mononuclear cells after centrifugation. So, this graft characteristic becomes an important consideration in heavily pretreated patients with renal compromise.

10.8.4 Nucleated Red Blood Cells

Nucleated red blood cells (NRBCs) can be present in substantial proportions in CB (Stevens et al. 2002). Most automated hematology analyzers enumerate NRBC and

WBC when performing counts, and the TNC (*total* nucleated cell) count of the CBU includes both populations. The presence of NRBCs in CBU TNC evaluation has two practical implications: firstly, NRBCs lyse more easily than WBC and may account for an overall lower cell recovery post-thaw. Secondly, there is a misconception that, because NRBCs are included in the TNC count, the engraftment ability of the CBU based on TNC may be "overestimated." The influence of the NRBC content on engraftment was evaluated by a retrospective study on 1112 recipients that received single CBU grafts provided by the NYBC. The evaluation showed that NRBC numbers correlated with CFU results indicating an overall bone marrow response and release of immature cells in the peripheral blood and, most importantly, they did not reduce the engraftment potential of the CBU (Stevens et al. 2002). So their presence, even in high numbers, does not imply a disadvantage for the CBU.

10.8.5 Hemoglobinopathy Screening

CBU hemoglobinopathy screening must utilize a methodology that distinguishes hemoglobins A, A2, S, C, F, and H. If there is a family history of hemoglobinopathy or if any hemoglobin types except HbA and HbF are detected, further testing is required. Units reported as normal or with "AF" hemoglobin pattern are acceptable. The presence of HbS (sickle cell hemoglobin) in addition to HbA and HbF indicates sickle cell trait. CBU homozygous for either sickle cell disease or thalassemia or heterozygous for both sickle cell and beta-thalassemia cannot be used for transplantation. Units heterozygous for either sickle cell trait or thalassemia can be used if other donor options are limited.

With current molecular testing assays for thalassemia, heterozygotes for α-thalassemia, evaluated because of elevated hemoglobin H on the screening assay or low mean corpuscular volume (MCV) in the complete blood count, are relatively frequent (Dobrila et al. 2016). Most are heterozygotes for a single α-globin gene deletion and therefore are "silent" carriers for α-thalassemia, so this molecular finding does not have clinical implications and there is no reason for CBU not to be used for transplantation (see Chap. 8).

10.8.6 ABO Blood Group

ABO blood group and Rh typing of the CBU are considered part of the identity testing. ABO incompatible, RBC-depleted CB units have not been shown to have a higher incidence of infusion reactions (Dahi et al. 2014b), probably because a large proportion of the RBCs lyse with the freezing and thawing procedure (not related to ABO incompatibility) and the patients are well hydrated. Although small studies showed some effect of ABO incompatibility on acute GvHD after CB transplants (Berglund et al. 2012), larger analyses have not confirmed this finding. There was no difference in incidence of acute or chronic GvHD in patients with malignant or nonmalignant diseases and CBU ABO incompatibility in the Minnesota studies

(Romee et al. 2013; Kudek et al. 2016; Damodar et al. 2017). Similarly no effect on GvHD or TRM was seen after single-unit CB grafts in a Japanese study (Konuma et al. 2013). Further, donor-recipient ABO matching did not influence RBC and platelet requirements after transplant (Solves et al. 2017). Based on these data, there appears to be no reason to include ABO/Rh type in CBU selection criteria.

10.8.7 Cord Blood Unit Cryopreservation Volume

Most automated CBU processing systems have a predefined, standardized final volume (e.g., 20 ml). In contrast, manually processed CBU may have variable final volumes. Cryoprotectant concentration and cooling rates during freezing procedures are important for the quality of the product, and these may vary, if the final volume is not standardized. CB banks report on the final cryopreservation volume of the CBU and whether the product is in one or two bags (or more). The method of CBU preparation for infusion has to be considered in regard to the CBU product volume. If albumin-dextran dilution is used and the bank recommends dilution seven- to eightfold, the infusion volume may be large for small pediatric patients (see Chaps. 6 and 9).

10.8.8 Bacteriology Screening

FDA and NetCord/FACT requirements mandate that CBU need to have negative bacterial and fungal cultures. CBU samples for bacteriology testing are obtained post-processing.

10.8.9 Infectious Disease Markers (IDM)

Infectious disease screening tests are performed on the maternal sample (collected within 7 days from CBU collection), as outlined by US FDA requirements (FDA Guidance for Industry 2007). Complete maternal IDM testing in a Clinical Laboratory Improvement Amendments (CLIA) certified laboratory is the standard. Of note, the testing requirements and approved screening assays change overtime, so stored CBU may not have all the currently required tests performed at the time of collection. Regulatory requirements and practice of medicine should guide the decisions about additional testing and acceptance of older CBU. Additional IDM requirements exist in other countries, and tests need to be performed prior to importing CBU. Information about stored maternal samples for future testing is important (see Chap. 8).

10.8.10 Donor Eligibility

CBU donor eligibility is based on the history and risk factors of the mother according to FDA guidelines and the results of the screening IDMs of the maternal sample

(FDA Guidance for Industry 2007). CBU from ineligible donors can be used for transplantation, based on FDA requirements of "urgent medical need" after evaluating the potential risk associated with the reason for ineligibility versus the potential benefit of the TNC and HLA match of the respective CBU relative to other graft options of the patient. This is further discussed in Chap. 8.

10.9 "Backup" Cord Blood Grafts

Many transplant centers have implemented the policy to have at least one backup CBU identified pre-transplant in the event that there are problems with unit shipping, thaw, infusion, or graft failure (Ponce et al. 2012). These backup units should have confirmatory HLA typing completed and need to be ready for shipment on the transplant day in case there are unexpected problems with the thawing of the graft. The NCBP, as well as many other domestic CB Banks, does not charge for CBU reservation as backup; however, several international banks may require fees if reserved CBU are not used.

10.10 Cord Blood Unit Selection for Unrelated Transplantation

Selection of CBU for transplantation remains a complex decision, and no algorithm "fits" all, since there are many considerations related to graft characteristics, the patient's disease, and clinical condition, as well as the treatment and type of transplant planned (Barker et al. 2011, 2017; Hough et al. 2016; Rocha 2016). While recommendations can be provided for selection of CBU for single or double unrelated grafts, transplant centers need to develop their own algorithms based on their specific studies as well as their results of post-thaw CBU evaluation (e.g., $CD34^+$ cell viability and $CD34^+$ cell recoveries) and patient outcomes (Barker et al. 2017). Further, selection of CBU to be used with novel expansion or homing strategies or with haploidentical grafts may be somewhat different, particularly regarding the TNC and $CD34^+$ cell doses.

10.11 Expert Opinion

With the growth of CB banking worldwide, it is important to evaluate domestic as well as international registries for each patient (Barker et al. 2011). The largest registry in the USA is the NMDP (National Marrow Donor Program, Be The Match Registry). Internationally, Bone Marrow Donors Worldwide (BMDW) is the largest unrelated donor and unrelated CBU registry reporting information from the USA and international CB banks (53 CB banks from 36 countries) (Bone Marrow Donors Worldwide n.d.).

For most transplant candidates, a search will display many potentially matched CBU. See Table 10.1.

10.12 Future Directions

The CB transplantation field has evolved tremendously over the last 25 years: the quality, safety, and efficacy of the unrelated CB grafts have improved significantly, and the transplant outcomes are comparable with those of unrelated adult volunteer donors. Improved CBU selection criteria and advanced clinical care, as well as better understanding of the supportive care needed for the CB recipients, have led to decreased rates of NRM and graft failure (Barker et al. 2017; Dahlberg and Milano 2016).

CB transplantation is well established in clinical practice, and several ongoing clinical trials aim to overcome some of the challenges, particularly the relatively low number of cells and the prolonged time to engraftment, by increasing the number of hematopoietic progenitor cells (ex vivo expansion studies) and/or their homing (reviewed in Ballen et al. 2013; Berglund et al. 2017). It is expected that these will also decrease the overall cost of CB transplantation, an aspect that is restricting the clinical use of CB grafts.

Besides the use in transplantation, several types of CB-derived cells are currently explored as treatments for viral infections, G*v*HD, malignancies, as well as in various studies of regenerative medicine: neurology, cardiology, endocrinology, and others (reviewed in Ballen et al. 2013; Dahlberg and Milano 2016). While these applications are under development, promising results are already noted for diseases with great impact on the general population, making the future of CB even more exciting.

Acknowledgments We thank the NYBC National Cord Blood Program staff who performs all the tasks needed to ensure the quality of the CBU and Dr. Pablo Rubinstein, Director of the National Cord Blood Program, for his support and constructive criticism. We are grateful to the obstetricians in the collaborating hospitals who support the National Cord Blood Program and to the mothers who generously donate their infant's cord blood. We also thank Professor Jon J. van Rood for his insight and support.

We thank the MSKCC hospital staff, clinical teams, unrelated search coordinators, and laboratories for excellent patient care, detailed evaluation of CBU searches, and post-thaw CBU studies.

References

Albano MS, Rothman W, Watanabe C, Gora A, Scaradavou A, Rubinstein P (2008) Hematopoietic colony forming unit: development of a high-throughput CFU assay strategy by the use of high-resolution digital images stored in a laboratory information system. Blood 112:2306. [abstract]

Albano MS, Stevens CE, Dobrila LN, Scaradavou A, Rubinstein P (2009) Colony-forming-unit (CFU) assay with high-resolution digital imaging: a reliable system for cord blood (CB) CFU evaluation. Biol Blood Marrow Transplant. 15:45. [abstract]

Albano MS, Rothman W, Scaradavou A, Blass DP, McMannis JD, Rubinstein P (2011) Automated counting of colony forming units (CFU): towards standardization of the measurement of potency in cord blood cell therapy products. Blood 118:485. [abstract]

Avery S, Shi W, Lubin M, Gonzales AM, Heller G, Castro-Malaspina H et al (2011) Influence of infused cell dose and HLA match on engraftment after double-unit cord blood allografts. Blood 117:3277–3285

Ballen K (2017) Umbilical cord blood transplantation: challenges and future directions. Stem Cells Transl Med. 6(5):1312

Ballen KK, Gluckman E, Broxmeyer HE (2013) Umbilical cord blood transplantation: the first 25 years and beyond. Blood 122:491–498

Barker JN, Scaradavou A (2011) The controversy of red blood cell-replete cord blood units. Blood 118:480. [Letter to Blood; Response]

Barker JN, Weisdorf DJ, DeFor TE, Blazar BR, Miller JS, Wagner JE (2003) Rapid and complete donor chimerism in adult recipients of unrelated donor umbilical cord blood transplantation after reduced-intensity conditioning. Blood 102:1915–1919

Barker JN, Weisdorf DJ, DeFor TE, Blazar BR, McGrave PB, Miller JS et al (2005) Transplantation of two partially HLA-matched umbilical cord blood units to enhance engraftment in adults with hematologic malignancy. Blood 105:1343–1347

Barker JN, Byam CE, Kernan NA, Lee SS, Hawke RM, Doshi KA et al (2010a) Availability of cord blood extends allogeneic hematopoietic stem cell transplant access to racial and ethnic minorities. Biol Blood Marrow Transplant. 16:1541–1548

Barker JN, Scaradavou A, Stevens CE (2010b) Combined effect of Total nucleated cell dose and HLA-match on transplant outcome in 1061 cord blood recipients with Hematological malignancies. Blood 115(9):1843

Barker JN, Byam C, Scaradavou A (2011) How I treat: the selection and acquisition of unrelated cord blood grafts. Blood 117:2332–2339

Barker JN, Kurtzberg J, Ballen K, Boo M, Brunstein C, Cutler C et al (2017) Optimal practices in unrelated donor cord blood transplantation for hematologic malignancies. Biol Blood Marrow Transplant. 23:882–896

Berglund S, Le Blanc K, Remberger M, Gertow J, Uzunel M, Svenberg P et al (2012) Factors with an impact on chimerism development and long-term survival after umbilical cord blood transplantation. Transplantation 94:1066–1074

Berglund S, Magalhaes I, Gaballa A, Vanherberghen B, Uhlin M (2017) Advances in umbilical cord blood cell therapy: the present and the future. Expert Opin Biol Ther 17:691–699

van Besien K, Childs R (2016) Haploidentical cord transplantation—the best of both worlds. Semin Hematol. 53:257–266

Bone Marrow Donors Worldwide (n.d.) http://www.bmdw.org

Broxmeyer HE, Srour EF, Hangoc G, Cooper S, Anderson SA, Bodine DM (2003) High-efficiency recovery of functional hematopoietic progenitor and stem cells from human cord blood cryopreserved for 15 years. Proc Natl Acad Sci U S A 100:645–650

Brunstein CG, Barker JN, Weisdorf DJ, DeFor TE, Miller JS, Blazar BR et al (2007) Umbilical cord blood transplantation after non-myeloablative conditioning: impact on transplant outcomes in 110 adults with hematological disease. Blood 110:3064–3070

Brunstein CG, Wagner JE, Weisdorf DJ, Cooley S, Noreen H, Barker JN et al (2009) Negative effect of KIR alloreactivity in recipients of umbilical cord blood transplant depends on transplantation conditioning intensity. Blood 113:5628–5634

Brunstein CG, Gutman JA, Weisdorf DJ et al (2010) Allogeneic hematopoietic cell transplantation for hematological malignancy: relative risks and benefits of double umbilical cord blood. Blood 116:4693–4699

Brunstein CG, Noreen H, DeFor TE, Maurer D, Miller JS, Wagner JE (2011) Anti-HLA antibodies in double umbilical cord blood transplantation. Biol Blood Marrow Transplant. 17:1704–1708

Brunstein C, Zhang MJ, Barker J, St Martin A, Bashey A, de Lima M et al (2017) The effect of inter-unit HLA matching in double umbilical cord blood transplantation of acute leukemia. Haematologica. 102:941–947

Burlingham WJ, Nelson LJ (2012) Microchimerism in cord blood: mother as anticancer drug. Proc Natl Acad Sci U S A 109:2190–2191

Chow R, Nademanee A, Rosenthal J, Karanes C, Jaing T-H, Graham M et al (2007) Analysis of hematopoietic cell transplants using plasma-depleted cord blood products that are not red cell reduced. Biol Blood Marrow Transplant. 13:1346–1357

Cunha R, Loiseau P, Ruggeri A, Sanz G, Michel G, Paolaiori A, Socié G et al (2014) Impact of HLA mismatch direction on outcomes after umbilical cord blood transplantation for hematological malignant disorders: a retrospective Eurocord-EBMT analysis. Bone Marrow Transplant. 49:24–29

Cutler C, Kim HT, Sun L, Sese D, Glotzbecker B, Armand P et al (2011) Donor-specific anti-HLA antibodies predict outcome in double umbilical cord blood transplantation. Blood 118:6691–6697

Dahi PB, Barone J, Devlin SM, Byam C, Lubin M, Ponce DM et al (2014a) Sustained donor engraftment in recipients of double-unit cord blood transplantation is possible despite donor-specific HLA-antibodies. Biol Blood Marrow Transplant. 20:787–793

Dahi PB, Lubin MN, Evans KL, Gonzales AMR, Schaible A, Tonon J et al (2014b) "No wash" albumin-dextran dilution for double-unit cord blood transplantation (DCBT) is safe with appropriate management and results in high rates of sustained donor engraftment. Biol Blood Marrow Transplant. 20:490–494

Dahlberg A, Milano F (2016) Cord blood transplantation: rewind to fast forward. Bone Marrow Transplant. https://doi.org/10.1038/bmt.2016.336

Damodar S, Snahley R, MacMillan M, Ustan C, Weisdorf D (2017) Donor-to-recipient ABO mismatch does not impact outcomes of allogeneic hematopoietic cell transplantation regardless of graft source. Biol Blood Marrow Transplant. 23:795–804

Dobrila L, Zhu T, Zamfir D, Tarnawski M, Ciubotariu R, Albano MS et al (2016) Detection of Hemoglobin (Hb) variants by HPLC screening in cord blood units (CBU) donated to the National Cord Blood Program (NCBP). Blood 128:2182. [abstract]

Eapen M, Rubinstein P, Zhang M-J, Stevens C, Kurtzberg J, Scaradavou A et al (2007) Outcomes of transplantation of unrelated donor umbilical cord blood and bone marrow in children with acute leukemia: a comparison study. Lancet 369:1947–1954

Eapen M, Rocha V, Sanz G, Scaradavou A, Zhang MJ, Arcese W et al (2010) Effect of graft source on unrelated donor haemopoietic stem-cell transplantation in adults with acute leukaemia: a retrospective analysis. Lancet Oncology 11:653–660

Eapen M, Klein PK, Sanz GF, Spellman S, Ruggeri A, Anasetti C et al (2011) Effect of donor-recipient HLA matching at HLA A, B, C, and DRB1 on outcomes after umbilical-cord blood transplantation for leukaemia and myelodysplastic syndrome: a retrospective analysis. Lancet 12:1214–1221

Eapen M, Klein PK, Ruggieri A, Spellman S, Lee SJ, Anasetti C et al (2014) Impact of allele-level HLA matching on outcomes after myeloablative single unit umbilical cord blood transplantation for hematologic malignancy. Blood 123:133–140

FDA Guidance for Industry (2007) Eligibility determination of donors of human cells, tissues, and cellular and tissue-based products (HCT/Ps). August 2007

FDA Guidance for Industry (2014) Biologics license applications for minimally manipulated, unrelated allogeneic placental/umbilical cord blood intended for hematopoietic and immunologic reconstitution in patients with disorders affecting the hematopoietic system. March 2014

Gluckman E, Rocha V (2009) Cord blood transplantation: state of the art. Hematologica. 94(4):451–454

Hough R, Danby R, Russell N, Marks D, Veys P, Shaw B et al (2016) Recommendations for a standard UK approach to incorporating umbilical cord blood into clinical transplantation practice: an update on cord blood unit selection, donor selection algorithms and conditioning protocols. Br J Haematol. 172:360–370

Keeney M, Chin-Yee I, Weir K, Popma J, Nayar R, Sutherland DR (1998) Single platform flow cytometric absolute CD34+ cell counts based on the ISHAGE guidelines. International Society of Hematotherapy and Graft Engineering. Cytometry 34:61–70

Konuma T, Kato S, Ooi J, Oiwa-Monna M, Ebihara Y, Mochizuki S et al (2013) Effect of ABO blood group incompatibility on the outcome of single-unit cord blood transplantation after myeloablative conditioning. Biol Blood Marrow Transplant 20:577–581. S1083-8791 [abstract]

Kudek MR, Shanley R, Zantek ND, McKenna DH, Smith AR, Miller WP (2016) Impact of graft-recipient ABO compatibility on outcomes after umbilical cord blood transplant for nonmalignant disease. Biol Blood Marrow Transplant. 22:2019–2024

Laughlin MJ, Barker J, Bambach B, Koc ON, Rizzieri DA, Wagner JE et al (2001) Hematopoietic engraftment and survival in adult recipients of umbilical cord blood from unrelated donors. N Engl J Med 344:1815–1822

Laughlin MJ, Eapen M, Rubinstein P, Wagner JE, Zhang MJ, Champlin RE, Stevens CE, Barker JN, Gale RP, Lazarus HM, Marks DI, van Rood JJ, Scaradavou A, Horowitz MM (2004) Outcomes after transplantation of cord blood or bone marrow from unrelated donors in adults with leukemia. N Engl J Med. 351:2265–2275

Matsuno N, Wake A, Uchida N, Ishiwata K, Aroaka H, Takagi S et al (2009) Impact of HLA disparity in the graft-versus-host direction on engraftment in adult patients receiving reduced-intensity cord blood transplantation. Blood 114:1689–1695

McCullough J, McKenna D, Kadidlo D, Maurer D, Noreen HJ, French K et al (2009) Mislabeled units of umbilical cord blood detected by a quality assurance program at the transplantation center. Blood 114(8):1684

Migliaccio AR, Adamson JW, Stevens CE, Dobrila NL, Carrier CM, Rubinstein P (2000) Cell dose and speed of engraftment in placental/umbilical cord blood transplantation: graft progenitor cell content is a better predictor than nucleated cell quantity. Blood 96:2717–2722

Milano F, Nelson LJ, Delaney C (2013) Fetal maternal immunity and antileukemia activity in cord-blood transplant recipients. Bone Marrow Transplant. 48:321–322

Milano F, Gooley T, Wood B, Woolfery A, Flowers ME, Doney K et al (2016) Cord-blood transplantation in patients with minimal residual disease. N Engl J Med. 375:944–953

Mitchell R, Wagner JE, Brunstein CG, Cao Q, McKenna DH, Lund TC et al (2015) Impact of long-term cryopreservation on single umbilical cord blood transplantation outcomes. Biol Blood Marrow Transplant. 21:50–54

Murphy A, McKenna D, McCullough J (2016) Cord blood banking and quality issues. Transfusion 56:645–652

Nawrot M, McKenna DH, Sumstad D, McMannis JD, Szczepiorkowski ZM, Belfield H et al (2011) Interlaboratory assessment of a novel colony-forming unit assay: a multicenter study by the cellular team of biomedical excellence for safer transfusion (BEST) collaborative. Transfusion 51:2001–2005

Nikiforow S, Li S, Snow K, Liney D, Kao GS, Haspel R et al (2017) Lack of impact of umbilical cord blood unit processing techniques on clinical outcomes in adult double cord blood transplant recipients. Cytotherapy. 19:272–284

NMDP (n.d.) Safety report to FDA and communication to transplant centers

Oran B, Shpall E (2013) Umbilical cord blood transplantation: a maturing technology. ASH educational program

Ottinger HD, Ferencik S, Beelen DW, Lindemann M, Peceny R, Elmaagacli AH et al (2003) Hematopoietic stem cell transplantation: contrasting the outcome of transplantations from HLA-identical siblings, partially HLA-mismatched related donors, and HLA matched unrelated donors. Blood 102:1131–1137

Page KM, Zhang L, Mendizabal A, Wease S, Carter S, Gentry T et al (2011) Total colony-forming units are a strong, independent predictor of neutrophil and platelet engraftment after unrelated umbilical cord blood transplantation: a single-center analysis of 435 cord blood transplants. Biol Blood Marrow Transplant. 17:1362–1374

Ponce DM, Lubin M, Gonzales AM, Byam C, Wells D, Ferrante R et al (2012) The use of back-up units to enhance the safety of unrelated donor cord blood transplantation. Biol Blood Marrow Transplant. 18:648–651

Prasad VK, Mendizabal A, Parikh SH, Szabolcs P, Driscoll TA, Page K et al (2008) Unrelated donor umbilical cord blood transplantation for inherited metabolic disorders in 159 pediatric patients from a single center: influence of cellular composition of the graft on transplantation outcomes. Blood 112:2979–2989

Purtill D, Smith KM, Tonon J, Evans KL, Lubin MN, Byam C et al (2013) Analysis of 402 cord blood units to assess factors influencing infused viable CD34+ cell dose: the critical determinant of engraftment. Blood 122:296. [abstract]

Querol S, Gomez SG, Pagliuca A, Torrabadella M, Madrigal JA (2010) Quality rather than quantity: the cord blood bank dilemma. Bone Marrow Transplant. 45:970–978

Reems JA, Hall KM, Gebru LH, Taber G, Rich IN (2008) Development of a novel assay to evaluate the functional potential of umbilical cord blood progenitors. Transfusion 48:620–628

Rocha V (2016) Umbilical cord blood cells from unrelated donor as an alternative source of hematopoietic stem cells for transplantation in children and adults. Seminars Hematol. 53:237–245

Rocha V, Wagner JE, Sobocinski KA, Klein JP, Zhang M-J, Horowitz MM et al (2000) Graft-versus-host disease in children who have received a cord blood or bone marrow transplant from an HLA-identical sibling. N Engl J Med. 342:1846–1854

Rocha V, Labopin M, Sanz G, Arcese W, Schwerdtfeger R, Bosi A et al (2004) Transplants of umbilical-cord blood or bone marrow from unrelated donors in adults with acute Leukemia. N Engl J Med. 351:2276–2285

Rocha V, Spellman S, Zhang MJ, Ruggeri A, Purtill D, Brady C et al (2012) Effect of HLA matching recipients to donor noninherited maternal antigens on outcomes after mismatched umbilical cord blood transplantation for hematologic malignancy. Biol Blood Marrow Transplant. 18:1890–1896

Rogriguez L, Garcia J, Querol S (2005) Predictive utility of an attached segment in the quality control of a cord blood graft. Biol Bone Marrow Transplant. 11:247–251

Romee R, Weisdorf DJ, Brunstein C, Wagner JE, Cao Q, Blazar BR et al (2013) Impact of ABO-mismatch on risk of GVHD after umbilical cord blood transplantation. Bone Marrow Transplant. 48:1046–1049

van Rood JJ, Oudshoorn M (2009) When selecting a HLA mismatched stem cell donor consider donor immune status. Curr Opin Immunol 21:1–6

van Rood JJ, Stevens CE, Schmits J, Carrier C, Carpenter C, Scaradavou A (2009) Re-exposure of cord blood to non-inherited maternal HLA antigens improves transplant outcome in hematological malignancies and might enhance its anti-leukemic effect. Proc Natl Acad Sci U S A 106:19952–19957

van Rood JJ, Scaradavou A, Stevens CE (2012) Indirect evidence that maternal microchimerism in cord blood mediates a graft-versus-leukemia effect in cord blood transplantation. Proc Natl Acad Sci U S A 109:2509–2514

Rubinstein P, Carrier C, Scaradavou A, Kurzberg J, Adamson J, Migliaccio AR et al (1998) Initial results of the placental/umbilical cord blood program for unrelated bone marrow reconstitution. N Engl J Med. 339:1565–1577

Ruggeri A, Rocha V, Masson E, Labopin M, Cunha R, Absi L et al (2013) Impact of donor-specific anti-HLA antibodies on graft failure and survival after reduced intensity conditioning-unrelated cord blood transplantation: a Eurocord, Société Francophone d'Histocompatibilité et d'Immunogénétique (SFHI) and Société Française de Greffe de Moelle et de Thérapie Cellulaire (SFGM-TC) analysis. Haematologica 98:1154–1160

Scaradavou A (2012) HLA-mismatched, noninherited maternal antigen-matched unrelated cord blood transplantations have superior survival: how HLA typing the cord blood donor's mother can move the field forward. Biol Blood Marrow Transplant. 18:1773–1775

Scaradavou A, Carrier C, Mollen N, Stevens C, Rubinstein P (1996) Detection of maternal DNA in placental/umbilical cord blood by locus-specific amplification of the non-inherited maternal HLA gene. Blood 88:1494–1500

Scaradavou A, Stevens CE, Dobrila L, Sung D, Rubinstein P (2007) "Age" of the cord blood (CB) unit: impact of long-term cryopreservation and storage on transplant outcome. Blood 110:2033. [abstract]

Scaradavou A, Smith KM, Hawke R, Schaible A, Abboud M, Kernan NA et al (2010) Cord blood units with low CD34+ cell viability have a low probability of engraftment after double unit transplantation. Biol Blood Marrow Transplant. 16:500–508

Scaradavou A, Brunstein CG, Eapen M, Le-Rademacher J, Barker JN, Chao N et al (2013) Double unit grafts successfully extend the application of umbilical cord blood transplantation on adults with acute leukemia. Blood 121:752–758

Scaradavou A, Dobrila L, Albano MS, Tarnawski M, Zhu T, Watanabe C et al (2016) Cord blood (CB) stability and potency evaluation: consistent, predictable recovery of hematopoietic progenitor cells (HPC) and high CD34+ cell viability in stored cord blood units (CBU) of the National Cord Blood Program (NCBP). Blood 128:2175. [abstract]

Shoulars K, Noldner P, Troy JD, Cheatham L, Parrish A, Page K et al (2016) Development and validation of a rapid, aldehyde dehydrogenase bright-based cord blood potency assay. Blood. 217:2346–2354

Solves P, Carpio N, Carretero C, Lorenzo JI, Sanz J, Gómez I et al (2017) ABO incompatibility does not influence transfusion requirements in patients undergoing single-unit umbilical cord blood transplantation. Bone Marrow Transplant. 52:394–399

Stevens CE, Gladstone J, Taylor PE, Scaradavou A, Migliaccio AR, Visser J et al (2002) Placental/umbilical cord blood for unrelated-donor bone marrow reconstitution: relevance of nucleated red blood cells. Blood 100:2662–2664

Stevens CE, Carrier C, Carpenter C, Sung D, Scaradavou A (2011) HLA mismatch direction in cord blood transplantation: impact on outcome and implications for cord blood unit selection. Blood 118:3969–3978

Takanashi M, Atsuta Y, Fujiwara K, Kodo H, Kai S, Sato H et al (2010) The impact of anti-HLA antibodies on unrelated cord blood transplantations. Blood 116:2839–2846

Van Rood JJ, Eemisse JG, van Leeuwen A (1958) Leukocyte antibodies in sera from pregnant women. Nature 181:1735–1736

Verneris MR, Brunstein CG, Barker J et al (2009) Relapse risk after umbilical cord blood transplantation: enhanced graft-versus-leukemia effect in recipienst of 2 units. Blood 114:4293–4299

Wagner JE (2016) Establishing the UCB graft potentiality. Blood 127:2272–2274

Wagner JE, Barker JN, DeFor TE, Baker KS, Blazar BR, Eide C et al (2002) Transplantation of unrelated donor umbilical cord blood in 102 patients with malignant and nonmalignant diseases: influence of CD34 cell dose and HLA disparity on treatment-related mortality and survival. Blood 100:1611–1618

Wagner JE, Eapen M, Carter SD, Wang Y, Schultz k WD et al (2014) One-unit versus two-unit cord-blood transplantation for hematologic cancers. N Engl J Med. 371:1685–1694

Willemze R, Rodrigues CA, Labopin M, Sanz G, Michel G, Socie G et al (2009) KIR-ligand incompatibility in the graft-versus-host direction improves outcomes after umbilical cord blood transplantation for acute leukemia. Leukemia 23:492–500

van den Zanden HG, van Rood JJ, Oudshoorn M, Bakker JN, Melis A, Brand A et al (2014) Noninherited maternal antigens identify acceptable HLA mismatches: benefits to patients and cost-effectiveness for cord blood banks. Biol Bone Marrow Transplant. 20:1791–1795

Cord Blood Graft Thawing

11

Ronit Reich-Slotky

11.1 Background

Cord blood (CB) units have been collected for the purpose of hematopoietic reconstitution since the 1980s. The first cord blood transplant was performed in Paris from an HLA-identical sibling to a patient with Fanconi's anemia (Gluckman et al. 1989). More than 25,000 cord blood transplants have been performed worldwide since then, with 2500 reported by the Center for International Blood and Marrow Transplant Research (CIBMTR) in 2015 (Butler and Menitove 2011; Pasquini and Zhu 2015). The advantage of using CB as an alternative cell source for hematopoietic progenitor cell (HPC) transplant is the higher HLA mismatch tolerance and the lower risk of graft-versus-host disease (G*v*HD) outcome in comparison with other hematopoietic progenitor cell (HPC) sources. CBU is also relatively easy to collect with no risk to the donor, and when a potential matched CB unit is recognized, it is a readily available for use.

Other allogeneic HPC sources, such as the bone marrow (BM) and peripheral blood (PB), are typically collected for an intendant recipient and are preferably infused fresh. Public cord blood banks (CBBs) collect CBs immediately after birth for future allogeneic use, typically for unknown recipient. For that reason CB units are cryopreserved for long-term storage, sometimes more than a decade. It is the combination of the need to cryopreserve, the potential dimethyl sulf oxide (DMSO) toxicity to both cells and patient, and the fact that CB units have relatively small cell dose that makes their preparation more challenging.

R. Reich-Slotky, Ph.D., M.Sc.
Department of Transfusion Medicine and Celluar Therapy, New York Presbyterian Hospital - Weill Cornell Medical Center, New York, NY, USA
e-mail: Ros9085@nyp.org

J. Schwartz, B.H. Shaz (eds.), *Best Practices in Processing and Storage for Hematopoietic Cell Transplantation*, Advances and Controversies in Hematopoietic Transplantation and Cell Therapy,
https://doi.org/10.1007/978-3-319-58949-7_11

11.2 The History of CB Processing and Cryopreservation

Broxmeyer and colleagues demonstrated in the late 1980s that CB cells could be obtained post-delivery from the cord and placenta and maintain their progenitor capacity after cryopreservation (Broxmeyer et al. 1989). In the early days, CBs were cryopreserved without removal of red blood cells (RBC) and plasma, resulting in significantly larger units. Due to their relatively larger volume, these units also contained higher DMSO volume, the molecule used for cryopreservation. Nowadays most CBBs remove both plasma and RBCs in a process that eliminates unnecessary cells and reduces the volume, thus reducing the final amount of DMSO used. This can be accomplished by either manual or automated methods using sedimentation with hydroxyethyl starch (HES) followed by plasma depletion. Some automated available technology includes PrepaCyte-CB Processing System (BioE, St Paul, MN) and Autopress Platform (Cesca Therapeutics, Rancho Cordova, CA). With these technologies the final volume of cryopreserved CB unit is typically ranging between 25 and 50 mL (Reich-Slotky et al. 2015; Young 2014).

11.3 DMSO Toxicity

To prevent cell death during cryopreservation due to formation of ice crystals, it is necessary to add a cryoprotectant. The standard cryoprotectant used for CB cryopreservation is DMSO, usually in a 10% final concentration. DMSO was originally used as an anti-inflammatory reagent, but in the 1990s, it was shown that DMSO can affect multiple organ systems with different toxicity levels, and its clinical use became controversial (Davis et al. 1990; Zambelli et al. 1998). To reduce the chance of side effects, the maximum recommended dose of DMSO is 1 mL/kg of recipient body weight (AABB et al. 2016). Due to CB unit's small volume, infusion-related adverse reactions associated with CB infusion are not as common as for other cryopreserved products, such as BM or PB (Chrysler et al. 2004). But reports of few severe, life-threatening adverse reactions associated with CB unit infusions prompted a review by the National Marrow Donor Program (NMDP) and the Food and Drug Administration (FDA), which found that in most investigated cases, at least one of the CB units infused was RBC replete (Choi et al. 2012). Based on their investigation, the NMDP and FDA provided recommendations for thawing and washing RBC-replete CB units (Miller 2009).

11.4 Unique CB Preparation Challenges

11.4.1 Unique Product with Small Cell Dose

Due to the nature of their collection, CBs are unique irreplaceable units. Compared to other HPC sources, CBs have a lower number of total nucleated cells (TNCs), and routine processing and cryopreservation can lead to an additional decrease in the number of TNCs and their viability. The established acceptable dose of HLA-matched CB for transplant is 2.5 million TNCs per kilogram (Migliaccio et al. 2000). Because of their limited cell dose, CBs have been used for many years mostly for transplant of pediatric patients, but new transplantation protocols have increased their use in adults, by using two CB units, expanded units, and/or engraftment-enhancing technologies (Ruggeri 2016). The relatively lower cell dose results in slower hematopoietic recover and higher susceptibility to infections and infection-related mortality than other HPC sources (Locatelli et al. 1999; Komanduri et al. 2007). The combination of limited cell dose and the nonavailability of the donor for additional collection increases the requirement to achieve high recovery of viable cells post processing.

11.4.2 Additional Variability Due to Different Manufacturers

Transplantation programs use CB units that have been collected, processed, and cryopreserved by family, public, and hybrid CBBs. Despite the effort to standardize CB processing, CBBs practice different manufacturing procedures, apply different quality criteria, and use different storage media and containers, thus increasing CB unit variability (Rubinstein et al. 1995; Alonso et al. 2001; Kurtzberg et al. 2005; Chow et al. 2011; Dazey et al. 2005; Takahashi et al. 2006). FDA cord blood licensing requirements are designed to assure quality and safety; currently seven CBBs are FDA licensed. Additionally, CB units may have been cryopreserved many years prior to current regulation and standardization.

Beside their manufacturing differences, each CBB develops and validates their own process for thawing and preparing units for transplantation, and although most CBBs use similar components for reconstitution and wash of CB units, their procedures may have small variation on factors such as component concentrations and dilution factors. These variations can present processing laboratories with additional challenges. Processing laboratories are required to develop validated process for preparation of cellular therapy products for transplantation and ensure that their technologists are trained and competent to perform the tasks. The variability in CBB manufacturing increases the complexity of developing one validated procedure for all CB units and requires that the laboratory will be ready to address unexpected deviations.

11.4.3 The Complexity of Preparing Cryopreserved Product for Transplantation

Cryopreservation can induce cell damage due to ice formation and dehydration (Mazur et al. 1972). Lovelock and Bishop reported the use of DMSO, a rapid penetrating molecule, for cryopreservation of living cells (Lovelock and Bishop 1959). If done properly, cryopreserved CB units can be stored in LN2 for extended time and maintain the HPC capacity (Broxmeyer et al. 2003; Mitchell et al. 2015). The same potential damaging factors that are present during cryopreservation pose potential harm during thaw. DMSO destabilizes the phospholipid membranes at higher temperatures, increasing the membrane leakage and cell destruction (Anchordoguy et al. 1992; Arakawa et al. 1990). Thus, thawing procedures of cryopreserved CB units should include steps to reduce growth of ice crystals and removal or dilution of high DMSO concentration, to decrease cell damage prior to product administration for transplantation (Mazur 2004). This requires highly trained technologists that can perform a complex process of an irreplaceable product for preconditioned patient.

11.5 Thawing Practices

Methods to process CB units should be selected to minimize cell losses, maintain cell viability, and prevent introduction of microbial contamination. Thawing should be done rapidly to avoid the possibility of recrystallization of any small intracellular ice nuclei, and steps should be taken to reduce DMSO concentration to prevent potential damaging osmotic swelling (Woods et al. 2000). Common thawing practices include bedside thaw, reconstitution and dilution with wash, and reconstitution and dilution without wash. Each method has advantages and disadvantages (Table 11.1), and the choice of which method to use depends on the qualification of the processing laboratory, the transplant program, and the CB unit itself.

Table 11.1 Comparison of different CB preparation methods

Method	Bedside thaw	Dilution (no wash)	Dilution and wash
Pros	• No processing • Minimal cell lose	• Controlled environment • Simple procedure • Minimal cell lose • Ability to sample and characterize • Long expiration time (~4 h)	• Controlled environment • Ability to sample and characterize • Removal of most DMSO and RBC • Long expiration time (~4 h) • Relatively small volume (25–100 mL)
Cons	• Uncontrolled environment • Increased DMSO toxicity • Limited ability to sample • Higher infusion-related AE • Short expiration time (~1 h)	• Relatively large volume • No reduction in RBC volume • No reduction in total DMSO volume and other potential toxic molecules (i.e., cytokines)	• Complex procedure • Cell loss • Risk of bag breakage

AE adverse event, *DMSO* dimethyl sulfoxide

11.5.1 Bedside Thaw

Direct thaw and administration of CB unit to the patient with no additional manipulation is commonly called bedside thaw because often it is performed in adjacent to the patient bedside, thus limiting the time between thaw and infusion and reducing the potential damage to the cells due to DMSO exposure.

To maintain the CB unit frozen, it should be delivered in a validated container that maintains the temperature below −135 °C. For the thaw process, units are typically placed in an outside plastic bag to prevent potential leaking in case of compromised bags. The wrapped unit is then placed in a water bath containing sterile water validated to maintain 37 °C temperature. The unit is removed from the water bath when all the ice crystals dissolve. Many laboratories use alternative validated dry warming devices, instead of a water bath for thawing. The advantage of these devices is that the units do not have to be submerged in water, a potential source of microbial contamination, and the device cleaning between products is easier. When the product is thawed, it is removed from the overwrap and infused.

Bedside thaw is an easy method that does not require highly trained technologists and can be performed by the nurses in the unit, if trained properly. Additionally, it results in little cell loss, especially if the empty bag is flushed with saline. Despite these advantages, the use of bedside thaw for CB units has fallen out of favor for many reasons. Cases of adverse events were reported for thaw and infusion of CB units without additional processing; many of them included at least one RBC-replete unit (Miller 2009). Once the product is thawed, any delay in infusion can further subject the cells to potential damage due to exposure to relatively high concentration of DMSO, without the benefit of the stabilizing effect of the protein- or colloid-based wash or dilution solution. Additional downside of this method is the fact that infusion preparation occurs outside of the controlled laboratory environment, preventing characterization and confirmation of product cellular content. If samples are obtained at the bedside for retrospective testing, the cells integrity and viability may be compromised due to DMSO exposure by the time they reach the laboratory. Some transplant programs still use bedside thaw for CB units, and despite the potential damage to the stem cells, the method did not prove to be associated with delayed engraftment. The Foundation for Accreditation of Cellular Therapy (FACT) standards and the National Marrow Donor Program (NMDP) protocol 10-CBA require the wash of RBC-replete CB units and strongly recommend the dilution or wash of RBC-depleted cords (also see Chaps. 6 and 7).

11.5.2 Thaw and Wash

Rubinstein and colleagues published in 1995 a thawing and washing method for CB units (Rubinstein et al. 1995). Their method was designed to address two major concerns: the potential risk to cell viability immediately after thaw and the need to remove toxic elements, such as DMSO, cell debris, and cytokines, and to reduce additional long-term cell damage and potential infusion adverse reaction. This method was used initially for products intended to children, who are more sensitive to DMSO toxicity due to their small body size, but eventually adopted for use in adult recipients as well. The method requires the immediate reconstitution of the thawed unit with equal volume of an isotonic solution containing protein source and colloids that help stabilize the membrane and reduce DMSO concentration, followed by further dilution with the same solution, a centrifugation step, and removal of most of the DMSO and hemolyzed RBCs (Rubinstein et al. 1995).

Over the years different cell processing laboratories and CBBs introduced minor variations to the original procedure, but most follow similar principles (Rubinstein et al. 1995). The unit is placed in an overwrap and thawed as described for bedside thaw. The thawed unit is slowly reconstituted with an equal volume of isotonic solution containing 5% dextran 40 and 2.5% human serum albumin (HSA) and allowed to equilibrate for 5 min. The unit is further diluted with the same solution to approximately 200 mL and centrifuged in 400 × *g* for 10 min. The supernatant is removed, and the cells are resuspended in the same solution, typically to 25–50 mL final volume.

Unlike bedside thaw, this process is done in the controlled laboratory environment with all critical steps being performed in the biological safety cabinet (BSC), allowing sampling for prospective testing such as viability and potency. The relative small volume of DMSO results in lower rates of adverse reactions (Foïs et al. 2007). This method was proven to reduce DMSO osmotic damage and maintain cell viability when compared to thaw alone. Additionally, the cell viability is stable for many hours, providing longer expiration time (Laroche et al. 2005; Chow et al. 2007). Despite all the benefits listed above, the procedure does carry some disadvantages. The wash and centrifugation steps are associated with cell loss. Laroche and colleagues reported an average of 82% TNC loss post wash (Laroche et al. 2005). Some have demonstrated that applying second centrifugation can recover some of the lost cells, but it increases the processing time and exposes the cells to additional damage. Bag punctures can occur due to inappropriate bag sealing or during cryopreservation, and the risk of bag breakage increases with the additional processing, such as centrifugation (Thyagarajan et al. 2008). Compromised bag can result in major cell loss, which can be critical for small units, and increases the potential of microbial contamination. Notably, the thaw and wash method does require the availability of highly trained and qualified laboratory technologists, and for small programs that perform few cord blood transplantations per year, this can be challenging.

11.5.3 Thaw and Dilution

As described above, the thaw and wash procedure has shown to sustain cell viability but may result in cell loss of an already small product. To overcome this problem, an alternative method that does not include the centrifugation step was developed (Barker et al. 2009). This method provides a simpler approach and takes advantage of the fact that most adults and larger pediatric patients can tolerate small volumes of DMSO with no significant adverse reactions. The harmful osmotic change is bypassed by diluting the thawed unit with a solution similar to the one described above (dextran/albumin) but without the additional centrifugation step and supernatant removal. The thawed cord is diluted with buffer. The CB unit to solution ratio ranges between 1:2 and 1:8 (Barker et al. 2009; Regan et al. 2010). Barker et al. reported that using this method on 54 consecutive CB unit transplants resulted in tolerable infusion reaction and high rates of sustainable engraftment. RBC-depleted cryopreserved unit was diluted at least 5.5 times to a median final volume of 200 mL (range, 200–500 mL); RBC-replete units were diluted at least 4 times their original volume to a median final volume of 400 mL (range, 400–535 mL). The reconstitution steps are performed in the laboratory and allow sampling for testing, and the progenitor cell viability and potency is compatible to the thaw and wash procedure (Regan et al. 2010).

This method is relatively straightforward and does not require complex training. It reduces the additional risk of bag breakage and cell loss while keeping the advantage of the stabilizing effect on cells provided by proteins and colloids. The disadvantage of this method is the infusion of DMSO and hemolyzed RBCs, and the overall unit large volume. The relatively large volume can increase the rates of DMSO-related adverse events as compared to the thaw and wash method and pose a risk to patients with renal deficiencies (Zambelli et al. 1998; Stroncek et al. 1991; Zenhäusern et al. 2000; Smith et al. 1987). Sixty-five percent of the patients described by Barker and colleagues experienced manageable infusion reaction, but few experienced transient renal insufficiency.

11.6 Expert Point of View

Many studies have shown that engraftment, transplant-related mortality, and overall survival after CB transplant correlate with variables such as donor-recipient HLA-match, nucleated cell dose, disease, and transplant regimens, but no clear relationship was found between the graft preparation method and transplant outcome (Migliaccio et al. 2000; Kurtzberg et al. 1996; Gluckman et al. 1997; Kurtzberg et al. 2008; Rocha et al. 2009; Wagner et al. 2002). In their early report, Kurtzberg et al. observed accelerated myeloid engraftment for washed units compared to bedside-thawed one, but the sample size was considerably small, and the GvHD prophylaxis regimen was also different between the groups (Kurtzberg et al. 1996). Other studies reported faster absolute neutrophil count (ANC) engraftment for non-washed CB units, but these were RBC-replete units with lower post thaw TNC dose (Chow et al. 2007). Most other studies did not demonstrate significant difference between the methods used (Regan et al. 2010; Nagamura-Inoue et al. 2003; Hahn et al. 2003).

Thaw and wash of CB is probably the most common method used, and, if done properly, it results in a product that can sustain cell viability for an extended time and results in lower rates of infusion adverse reactions. But additional factor should be considered by transplant programs before choosing the best preparation method. These factors include the transplant setting, the availability of trained staff, and the CB manufacturer.

Small adult transplant programs with limited availability of highly trained laboratory staff may choose to use the bedside method or the thaw and dilution method. Both methods do not reduce the DMSO volume but are simple and require no or simple processing steps. Programs that do not have processing laboratory on site and use outside services that are within acceptable distance, or programs that serve pediatric patients, should use the thaw and wash method. This method removes most of the DMSO and other toxins and sustains cell viability for extended time, thus allowing short-distance shipping from remote processing facility.

Although most CBBs use similar approaches to collect, process, and cryopreserve CB units, there are differences in production methods that contribute to final product variations. Every CBB develops and validates procedures for handling their products. The advantage of using a recommended CBB method for each CB is that it was validated for the specific production method and it is probably optimized for the manufacturer product. It is also useful for small programs that do not typically process CBs for transplant but suddenly have to prepare one. In this scenario, if the CBB recommended method is used, there is no need to perform a full processing validation, and as long as the staff is trained to perform similar procedures, the method can be used. Still many processing facilities use their own validated procedure for preparing CBs for transplant regardless of the CB manufacturer recommended method. Using a uniform method for all CBs eases training and process control, while using slightly different methods each time can be confusing for laboratory technologists, can add processing variability, and complicates document control. Additionally, components that have been validated by CBB might be unavailable at the time of CB use. In 2014 there was a national shortage in dextran 40 in the USA. This forced many laboratories to either start using lower-grade reagents or design a new wash solution (Reich-Slotky et al. 2015).

11.7 Future Direction

Future efforts should be directed to improve and standardize manufacturing of CB units. Better understanding of the mechanism of cell damage by cryopreservation will help optimize the process. This would include investigating parameters such as sample harvest and preparation, optimal cell concentration, additives used in the process, and freezing curves. Additionally, development of alternative, less toxic cryoprotectants will reduce the need to wash cells and will result in more stable products with lower toxicity. There are ongoing attempts to develop alternative cryoprotecting molecules either without or with reduced DMSO concentration (Bakken et al. 2003; Zeisberger et al. 2011). Disaccharide molecules such as trehalose and sucrose were shown to maintain membrane and protein integrity during cryopreservation, and their combination with DMSO concentration as low as 2.5% in cryopreservation of CB units was shown to be compatible with the traditional

10% DMSO concentration (Woods et al. 2000; Rodrigues et al. 2008; Zhang et al. 2003). Recent publication by Svalgaard and colleagues explored the use of low-molecular-weight carbohydrate Pentaisomaltose (PIM) as an alternative to DMSO in cryopreservation of PBHC. They demonstrated that progenitor cell recovery and potency was similar between PBHC products cryopreserved with PIM and DMSO (Svalgaard et al. 2016).

Automated washing systems can provide a uniform method that is easy to teach and operate and can reduce introduction of microbial contamination during processing. In the last few years, few devices were developed to provide close systems for washing CB units and other HPC products. Different automated devices were shown by few groups to result in high cell recovery and viable progenitor cells (Rodríguez et al. 2004; Perotti et al. 2004; Scerpa et al. 2011; Sánchez-Salinas et al. 2012; Zinno et al. 2011).

Standardization of CB unit manufacturing by CBB worldwide can reduce product variability and help develop a uniform post thaw processing method, and efforts should be made to make CB processing as efficient and uniform as possible. The use of automated system by CBB for processing of CBs results in higher TNC and $CD34^+$ cell recovery (Lapierre et al. 2007; Solves et al. 2009). On the other hand, different processing methods result in different cell type recoveries; therefore, optimizing the method to the intended use of the cord may be considered (Basford et al. 2010). As the cellular therapy field changes and the use of CB expands beyond hematopoietic reconstitution, the manufacturing and processing of CBs will need to develop and adjust accordingly.

References

AABB AAoTB, American Red Cross, American Society for Blood and Marrow, Transplantation ASfA, America's Blood Centers, College of American Pathologists, Cord Blood Association, Foundation for the Accreditation of, Cellular Therapy I, International NetCord Foundation, International Society for Cellular Therapy, JACIE Accreditation Office, Program NMD (2016) Circular of information for the use of cellular therapy products. AABB, Bethesda, MD

Alonso JM, Regan DM, Johnson CE et al (2001) A simple and reliable procedure for cord blood banking, processing, and freezing: St Louis and Ohio Cord Blood Bank experiences. Cytotherapy 3(6):429–433

Anchordoguy TJ, Carpenter JF, Crowe JH, Crowe LM (1992) Temperature-dependent perturbation of phospholipid bilayers by dimethyl sulfoxide. Biochim Biophys Acta 1104(1):117–122

Arakawa T, Carpenter JF, Kita YA, Crowe JH (1990) The basis for toxicity of certain cryoprotectants: a hypothesis. Cryobiology 27:401–415

Bakken AM, Bruserud O, Abrahamsen JF (2003) No differences in colony formation of peripheral blood stem cells frozen with 5% or 10% dimethyl sulfoxide. J Hematother Stem Cell Res 12(3):351–358

Barker JN, Abboud M, Rice RD et al (2009) A "no-wash" albumin-dextran dilution strategy for cord blood unit thaw: high rate of engraftment and a low incidence of serious infusion reactions. Biol Blood Marrow Transplant 15(12):1596–1602

Basford C, Forraz N, Habibollah S, Hanger K, McGuckin C (2010) The cord blood separation league table: a comparison of the major clinical grade harvesting techniques for cord blood stem cells. Int J Stem Cells 3(1):32–45

Broxmeyer HE, Douglas GW, Hangoc G et al (1989) Human umbilical cord blood as a potential source of transplantable hematopoietic stem/progenitor cells. Proc Natl Acad Sci U S A 86(10):3828–3832

Broxmeyer HE, Srour EF, Hangoc G, Cooper S, Anderson SA, Bodine DM (2003) High-efficiency recovery of functional hematopoietic progenitor and stem cells from human cord blood cryopreserved for 15 years. Proc Natl Acad Sci U S A 100(2):645–650

Butler MG, Menitove JE (2011) Umbilical cord blood banking: an update. J Assist Reprod Genet 28(8):669–676

Choi S, Hoffmann S, Cooling L (2012) Another case of acute cardiopulmonary toxicity with cord blood infusion: is dextran the culprit? Transfusion 52(1):207–208

Chow R, Nademanee A, Rosenthal J et al (2007) Analysis of hematopoietic cell transplants using plasma-depleted cord blood products that are not red blood cell reduced. Biol Blood Marrow Transplant 13(11):1346–1357

Chow R, Lin A, Tonai R et al (2011) Cell recovery comparison between plasma depletion/reduction- and red cell reduction-processing of umbilical cord blood. Cytotherapy 13(9):1105–1119

Chrysler G, McKenna D, Scheierman T et al (2004) Umbilical cord blood banking. In: Broxmeyer HE (ed) Cord blood: biology, immunology, banking and clinical transplantation. American Association of Blood Banks, Bethesda, MD, pp 219–257

Davis JM, Rowley SD, Braine HG, Piantadosi S, Santos GW (1990) Clinical toxicity of cryopreserved bone marrow graft infusion. Blood 75(3):781–786

Dazey B, Duchez P, Letellier C, Vezon G, Ivanovic Z, Network FCB (2005) Cord blood processing by using a standard manual technique and automated closed system "Sepax" (Kit CS-530). Stem Cells Dev 14(1):6–10

Foïs E, Desmartin M, Benhamida S et al (2007) Recovery, viability and clinical toxicity of thawed and washed haematopoietic progenitor cells: analysis of 952 autologous peripheral blood stem cell transplantations. Bone Marrow Transplant 40(9):831–835

Gluckman E, Broxmeyer HA, Auerbach AD et al (1989) Hematopoietic reconstitution in a patient with Fanconi's anemia by means of umbilical-cord blood from an HLA-identical sibling. N Engl J Med 321(17):1174–1178

Gluckman E, Rocha V, Boyer-Chammard A et al (1997) Outcome of cord-blood transplantation from related and unrelated donors. Eurocord Transplant Group and the European Blood and Marrow Transplantation Group. N Engl J Med 337(6):373–381

Hahn T, Bunworasate U, George MC et al (2003) Use of nonvolume-reduced (unmanipulated after thawing) umbilical cord blood stem cells for allogeneic transplantation results in safe engraftment. Bone Marrow Transplant 32(2):145–150

Komanduri KV, St John LS, de Lima M et al (2007) Delayed immune reconstitution after cord blood transplantation is characterized by impaired thymopoiesis and late memory T-cell skewing. Blood 110(13):4543–4551

Kurtzberg J, Laughlin M, Graham ML et al (1996) Placental blood as a source of hematopoietic stem cells for transplantation into unrelated recipients. N Engl J Med 335(3):157–166

Kurtzberg J, Cairo MS, Fraser JK et al (2005) Results of the cord blood transplantation (COBLT) study unrelated donor banking program. Transfusion 45(6):842–855

Kurtzberg J, Prasad VK, Carter SL et al (2008) Results of the Cord Blood Transplantation Study (COBLT): clinical outcomes of unrelated donor umbilical cord blood transplantation in pediatric patients with hematologic malignancies. Blood 112(10):4318–4327

Lapierre V, Pellegrini N, Bardey I et al (2007) Cord blood volume reduction using an automated system (Sepax) vs. a semi-automated system (Optipress II) and a manual method (hydroxyethyl starch sedimentation) for routine cord blood banking: a comparative study. Cytotherapy 9(2):165–169

Laroche V, McKenna DH, Moroff G, Schierman T, Kadidlo D, McCullough J (2005) Cell loss and recovery in umbilical cord blood processing: a comparison of postthaw and postwash samples. Transfusion 45(12):1909–1916

Locatelli F, Rocha V, Chastang C et al (1999) Factors associated with outcome after cord blood transplantation in children with acute leukemia. Eurocord-Cord Blood Transplant Group. Blood 93(11):3662–3671

Lovelock JE, Bishop MW (1959) Prevention of freezing damage to living cells by dimethyl sulphoxide. Nature 183(4672):1394–1395

Mazur P (2004) Principles of cryobiology. In: Fuller BJLN, Benson E (eds) Life in the frozen state. CRC, Boca Raton, FL, pp 3–66

Mazur P, Leibo SP, Chu EH (1972) A two-factor hypothesis of freezing injury. Evidence from Chinese hamster tissue-culture cells. Exp Cell Res 71(2):345–355

Migliaccio AR, Adamson JW, Stevens CE, Dobrila NL, Carrier CM, Rubinstein P (2000) Cell dose and speed of engraftment in placental/umbilical cord blood transplantation: graft progenitor cell content is a better predictor than nucleated cell quantity. Blood 96(8):2717–2722

Miller JA (2009) Centralized cord blood registry to facilitate allogeneic, unrelated cord blood transplantation. National Marrow Donor Program, Minneapolis, MN

Mitchell R, Wagner JE, Brunstein CG et al (2015) Impact of long-term cryopreservation on single umbilical cord blood transplantation outcomes. Biol Blood Marrow Transplant 21(1):50–54

Nagamura-Inoue T, Shioya M, Sugo M et al (2003) Wash-out of DMSO does not improve the speed of engraftment of cord blood transplantation: follow-up of 46 adult patients with units shipped from a single cord blood bank. Transfusion 43(9):1285–1295

Pasquini M, Zhu X (2015) Current uses and outcomes of hematopoietic stem cell transplantation: CIBMTR summary slides. http://www.cibmtr.org

Perotti CG, Del Fante C, Viarengo G et al (2004) A new automated cell washer device for thawed cord blood units. Transfusion 44(6):900–906

Regan DM, Wofford JD, Wall DA (2010) Comparison of cord blood thawing methods on cell recovery, potency, and infusion. Transfusion 50(12):2670–2675

Reich-Slotky R, Bachegowda LS, Ancharski M et al (2015) How we handled the dextran shortage: an alternative washing or dilution solution for cord blood infusions. Transfusion 55(6):1147–1153

Rocha V, Gluckman E, Group E-NraEBaMT (2009) Improving outcomes of cord blood transplantation: HLA matching, cell dose and other graft- and transplantation-related factors. Br J Haematol 147(2):262–274

Rodrigues JP, Paraguassú-Braga FH, Carvalho L, Abdelhay E, Bouzas LF, Porto LC (2008) Evaluation of trehalose and sucrose as cryoprotectants for hematopoietic stem cells of umbilical cord blood. Cryobiology 56(2):144–151

Rodríguez L, Azqueta C, Azzalin S, García J, Querol S (2004) Washing of cord blood grafts after thawing: high cell recovery using an automated and closed system. Vox Sang 87(3):165–172

Rubinstein P, Dobrila L, Rosenfield RE et al (1995) Processing and cryopreservation of placental/umbilical cord blood for unrelated bone marrow reconstitution. Proc Natl Acad Sci U S A 92(22):10119–10122

Ruggeri A (2016) Alternative donors: cord blood for adults. Semin Hematol 53(2):65–73

Sánchez-Salinas A, Cabañas-Perianes V, Blanquer M et al (2012) An automatic wash method for dimethyl sulfoxide removal in autologous hematopoietic stem cell transplantation decreases the adverse effects related to infusion. Transfusion 52(11):2382–2386

Scerpa MC, Daniele N, Landi F et al (2011) Automated washing of human progenitor cells: evaluation of apoptosis and cell necrosis. Transfus Med 21(6):402–407

Smith DM, Weisenburger DD, Bierman P, Kessinger A, Vaughan WP, Armitage JO (1987) Acute renal failure associated with autologous bone marrow transplantation. Bone Marrow Transplant 2(2):195–201

Solves P, Mirabet V, Blanquer A et al (2009) A new automatic device for routine cord blood banking: critical analysis of different volume reduction methodologies. Cytotherapy 11(8):1101–1107

Stroncek DF, Fautsch SK, Lasky LC, Hurd DD, Ramsay NK, McCullough J (1991) Adverse reactions in patients transfused with cryopreserved marrow. Transfusion 31(6):521–526

Svalgaard JD, Haastrup EK, Reckzeh K et al (2016) Low-molecular-weight carbohydrate Pentaisomaltose may replace dimethyl sulfoxide as a safer cryoprotectant for cryopreservation of peripheral blood stem cells. Transfusion 56(5):1088–1095

Takahashi TA, Rebulla P, Armitage S et al (2006) Multi-laboratory evaluation of procedures for reducing the volume of cord blood: influence on cell recoveries. Cytotherapy 8(3):254–264

Thyagarajan B, Berger M, Sumstad D, McKenna DH (2008) Loss of integrity of umbilical cord blood unit freezing bags: description and consequences. Transfusion 48(6):1138–1142

Wagner JE, Barker JN, DeFor TE et al (2002) Transplantation of unrelated donor umbilical cord blood in 102 patients with malignant and nonmalignant diseases: influence of CD34 cell dose and HLA disparity on treatment-related mortality and survival. Blood 100(5):1611–1618

Woods EJ, Liu J, Derrow CW, Smith FO, Williams DA, Critser JK (2000) Osmometric and permeability characteristics of human placental/umbilical cord blood CD34+ cells and their application to cryopreservation. J Hematother Stem Cell Res 9(2):161–173

Young W (2014) Plasma-depleted versus red cell-reduced umbilical cord blood. Cell Transplant 23(4–5):407–415

Zambelli A, Poggi G, Da Prada G et al (1998) Clinical toxicity of cryopreserved circulating progenitor cells infusion. Anticancer Res 18(6B):4705–4708

Zeisberger SM, Schulz JC, Mairhofer M et al (2011) Biological and physicochemical characterization of a serum- and xeno-free chemically defined cryopreservation procedure for adult human progenitor cells. Cell Transplant 20(8):1241–1257

Zenhäusern R, Tobler A, Leoncini L, Hess OM, Ferrari P (2000) Fatal cardiac arrhythmia after infusion of dimethyl sulfoxide-cryopreserved hematopoietic stem cells in a patient with severe primary cardiac amyloidosis and end-stage renal failure. Ann Hematol 79(9):523–526

Zhang XB, Li K, Yau KH et al (2003) Trehalose ameliorates the cryopreservation of cord blood in a preclinical system and increases the recovery of CFUs, long-term culture-initiating cells, and nonobese diabetic-SCID repopulating cells. Transfusion 43(2):265–272

Zinno F, Landi F, Scerpa MC et al (2011) Processing of hematopoietic stem cells from peripheral blood before cryopreservation: use of a closed automated system. Transfusion 51(12):2656–2663

Hematopoietic Graft Handling During Transportation

12

David Ming-Hung Lin, Jeannene Marie Gibbons, Alexander Thomas Gallacher, and Rebecca Haley

12.1 Introduction

The cell source for hematopoietic cell transplantation (HCT) can be autologous, related allogeneic, or unrelated allogeneic. Autologous cell therapy (CT) and related allogeneic CD34⁺ cell products are often collected and processed in the same facility as the transplant center. This is not the case, however, for unrelated donor cord blood, peripheral blood, or bone marrow transplantation that are facilitated by registries—such as the National Marrow Donor Program (NMDP) and the World Marrow Donor Association (WMDA)—that are involved in the public exchange of these allogeneic CT products worldwide. Non-cryopreserved and cryopreserved allogeneic CT products are, therefore, frequently transferred on public roads as well as on aircrafts to geographically distant facilities. Since the infusion is usually scheduled within 48–72 h after collection (for non-cryopreserved CT products) or after receipt at the transplant center (for cryopreserved CT products), this process mandates complex coordination by highly trained personnel. The process of transferring CT products is tightly regulated by the Food and Drug Administration (FDA), Department of Transportation (DOT), International Air Transport Association (IATA), International

D.M.-H. Lin, M.D., M.H.A. (✉)
Apheresis Services, NMDP Apheresis Center, Coord Blood Services, Bloodworks, Seattle, WA, USA
e-mail: dlin@bloodworksnw.org

J.M. Gibbons, B.S. • A.T. Gallacher, B.S.
Cord Blood Services, Bloodworks, Seattle, WA, USA
e-mail: jeanneneg@bloodworksnw.org; alexga@bloodworksnw.org

R. Haley, M.D.
Blood Services, Cord Blood Services, Cell Processing Lab and NMDP Apheresis Center, Bloodworks, Seattle, WA, USA
e-mail: beckyh@bloodworksnw.org

J. Schwartz, B.H. Shaz (eds.), *Best Practices in Processing and Storage for Hematopoietic Cell Transplantation*, Advances and Controversies in Hematopoietic Transplantation and Cell Therapy,
https://doi.org/10.1007/978-3-319-58949-7_12

Civil Aviation Organization (ICAO), AABB (formerly known as the American Association of Blood Banks), and Foundation for the Accreditation of Cellular Therapy (FACT). The regulations that must be followed depend on the hazardous material classification of the biological and cryogenic substances in the transfer container. The requirements for continuous temperature monitoring and the procedures for packaging, labeling, and documentation are all designed to maintain the integrity of the CT product while protecting the health and safety of personnel involved in the transfer process. It is essential to clearly document the chain of custody as the CT product is transferred from the cosigner (transfer facility) to the consignee (receiving facility) via the courier. Upon receipt, trained personnel at the receiving facility should promptly follow the instructions for opening the container and inspecting the CT product as well as make a decision to accept, reject, or quarantine the CT product.

12.2 Transferring Cell Therapy Products for Hematopoietic Cell Transplantation

Transport and *shipping* refer to the physical act of transferring CT products within or between facilities (The Foundation for the Accreditation of Cellular Therapy (FACT) and the Joint Accreditation Committee ISCT and EBMT 2015). These terms are not synonymous, however, and should not be used interchangeably. During transportation, the CT product "does not leave the control" of trained personnel such as a courier. In contrast, during shipping, the CT product "leaves the control" of trained personnel. In this chapter, for the sake of simplicity, we will use "transfer" to refer to both transport and shipping.

Non-cryopreserved CT products are transferred in a thermally insulated container to ensure the maintenance of temperatures within the acceptable range for the expected duration of the transfer. This is required by the Foundation for the Accreditation of Cellular Therapy (FACT) when the intended recipient has *already received* myeloablative conditioning (The Foundation for the Accreditation of Cellular Therapy (FACT) and the Joint Accreditation Committee ISCT and EBMT 2015). Cryopreserved CT products are transferred in a dry shipper and stored at the transplant center *before* the intended recipient has received myeloablative conditioning.

12.3 Electronic Data Loggers

During the transfer of CT products, continuous *temperature monitoring devices* (TMDs) are required by both FACT and the AABB (The Foundation for the Accreditation of Cellular Therapy (FACT) and the Joint Accreditation Committee ISCT and EBMT 2015; AABB 2015). Temperature extremes due to seasonal variations have been shown to be detrimental to the viability of mononuclear cells in non-cryopreserved CT products transferred in validated containers (Olson et al. 2011). For cryopreserved CT products, prolonged latency at the eutectic transition point—where liquids transition to a crystalline phase with the release of fusion heat—is damaging to cell survivability (Yang et al. 2011; Donaldson et al. 1996).

A variety of electronic data loggers are available for thermally insulated containers (e.g., Marathon TMD) and dry shippers (e.g., ShipsLog TMD and Libero TMD). TMDs shown in Fig. 12.1 are currently being, or have previously been, used by our institution's processing facility. Data loggers equipped with a visual temperature display are preferred. If a visual temperature display is not available, the receiving facility can request a temperature tracing once the data logger has been returned to the transfer facility. Examples of acceptable and unacceptable temperature tracings are shown in Figs. 12.2 and 12.3, respectively.

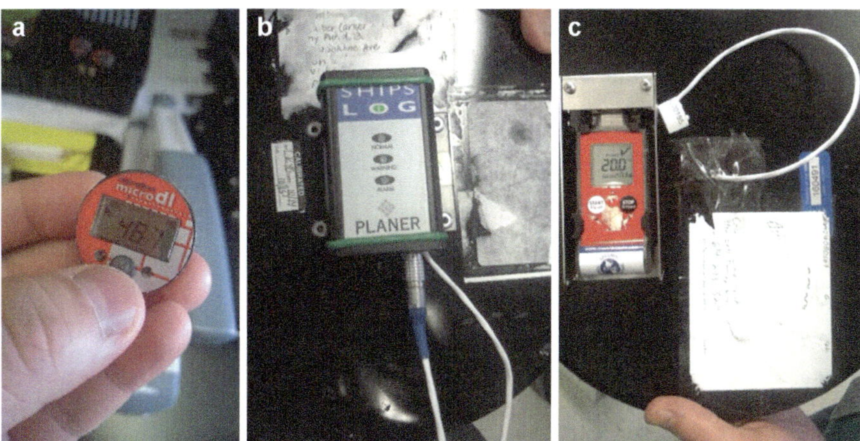

Fig. 12.1 Examples of continuous temperature monitoring devices: (**a**) Marathon micro-DL8, (**b**) Planer ShipsLog, and (**c**) Libero

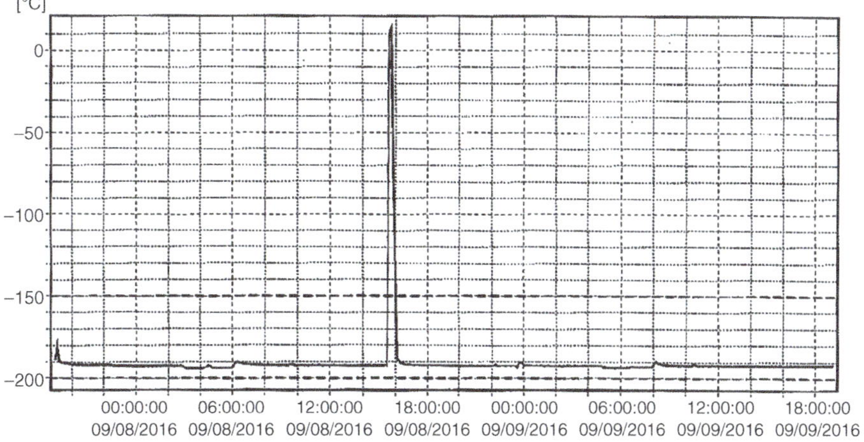

Fig. 12.2 Example of an acceptable temperature tracing downloaded from TMD. The tracing shows that the CT product is maintained at less than −150 °C until the dry shipper was opened and closed by the transplant center around 17:00 on September 8, 2016

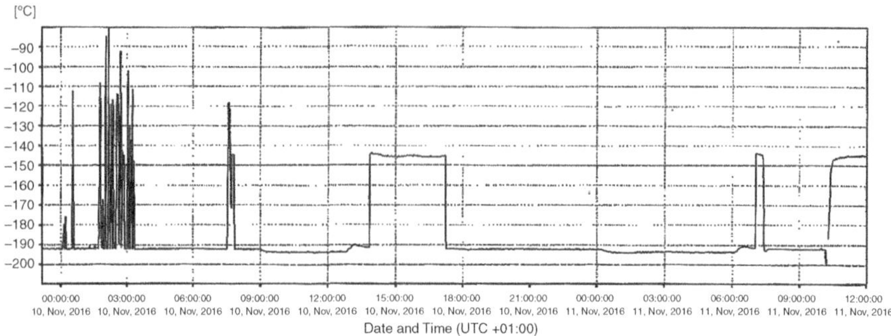

Fig. 12.3 Example of an unacceptable tracing downloaded from an electronic temperature monitoring device (TMD). **From left to right**, the tracing shows unusual temperature spikes, followed by a prolonged plateau and a brief plateau, and then a short duration period where TMD failed to sense and capture the temperature. The conclusion of the investigation was that the tracing was erroneous due to a failing TMD. No mishandling during shipment or tampering of the dry shipper was discovered

12.4 Transfer Containers

12.4.1 Transferring Non-cryopreserved CT Products

To prevent leakage, non-cryopreserved CT products and their accompanying samples are first placed in a sealed secondary container, such as resealable plastic bag, with surrounding absorbent material in sufficient quantity to absorb the entire content. During transfer, the product and samples are together held in a thermally insulated outer container that is validated to ensure the maintenance of temperatures within the acceptable range—either at room temperature, typically 18–24 °C, or cooled to 2–8 °C using cold packs—for the expected duration of transfer (AABB 2015). The container should also withstand leakage of contents, impact shocks, pressure changes, temperature changes, puncture, and other conditions incident to handling during shipping. These handling activities are tested during container validation and may include riding in a transport vehicle, dropping the container from the height of a loading platform, falling from a hand truck, or similar activities (The Foundation for the Accreditation of Cellular Therapy (FACT) and the Joint Accreditation Committee ISCT and EBMT 2015).

Each institution defines its own validated transfer conditions, including temperature. For freshly collected hematopoietic progenitor cell (HPC) apheresis products, Antonenas and coworkers (2006) reported that the optimal temperature for maintaining the $CD34^{+}$ viability is at refrigerated temperatures (2–8 °C). This refrigerated temperature condition is what the NMDP requires—unless room temperature is specifically requested by the transplant center—for the transfer of allogeneic HPC apheresis products. On the other hand, for newly collected HPC cord blood products, the optimal transit temperatures are not as well established. This leaves each facility to define and validate acceptable transfer temperature limits. For example, a validation study by Wada and coworkers (2004) reported that the viability of cord blood units (CBU) shipped at "ambient" temperature is expected to decrease by 1% every 4 h.

12.4.2 Physical and Chemical Properties of Liquid Nitrogen

Liquid N2 is a nonflammable substance that boils at −196 °C. One liter of liquid N2, when completely transitioned to vapor phase, will expand into 0.7 m^3 of N2 gas at 1 atmosphere of pressure and 21 °C. In a poorly ventilated space, vaporized liquid N2 will enrich the N2 content of air while depleting its oxygen content. Odorless and colorless vapor N2 is a dangerous asphyxiant; therefore, oxygen depletion should be monitored in areas where liquid N2 is stored (Fig. 12.4a). As always, appropriate personal protective equipment (PPE)—such as insulated gloves, safety glasses, and close-toed shoes—should be worn at all times when handling liquid N2-filled containers.

12.4.3 Transferring Cryopreserved CT Products

Cryopreserved CT products frozen and stored in nitrogen (N2) vapor must be shipped in a validated, vacuum-insulated dry shipper. The walls of dry shippers contain a hydrophobic absorbent material so that when charged according to the manufacturer's instructions, the dry shipper releases vapor N2 at a rate that is able to maintain the cryogenic temperature at less than −150 °C for a required period of time of at least 48 h beyond the expected time of delivery at the receiving facility. The expected cryogenic hold time can be calculated using the charged and empty weight differential of the dry shipper (measured in pounds), the normal evaporation rate in upright position (expressed in liters per day), and a unit conversion of N2 gas (i.e., 0.5606 L of N2 per pound of N2) measured at 1 atmosphere of pressure and 21 °C. During transfer, the dry shipper should always be kept in an upright position so that the vapor N2 sinks to the bottom of the cryogenic chamber. If the dry shipper is laid on its side or positioned upside down, vapor N2 would escape the cryogenic chamber (accelerated nitrogen evaporation rate) and greatly reduce the cryogenic hold time:

$$\text{Hold time}(\text{days}) = \frac{(\text{Charged} - \text{Empty Dry Shipper Weight}) \times (0.5606)}{\text{Normal Evaporation Rate in Upright Position}}$$

Before being placed into service, dry shippers must be inspected and qualified. For example, inspecting the outside of the dry shipper for excessive condensation is a visual clue that the vacuum insulation may be compromised. The cryogenic chamber is filled with liquid N2 and charged according to the manufacturer's instructions (Fig. 12.4b). An example of instructions on charging a dry shipper is provided in Table 12.1. Next, the dry shipper must be carefully and completely emptied of

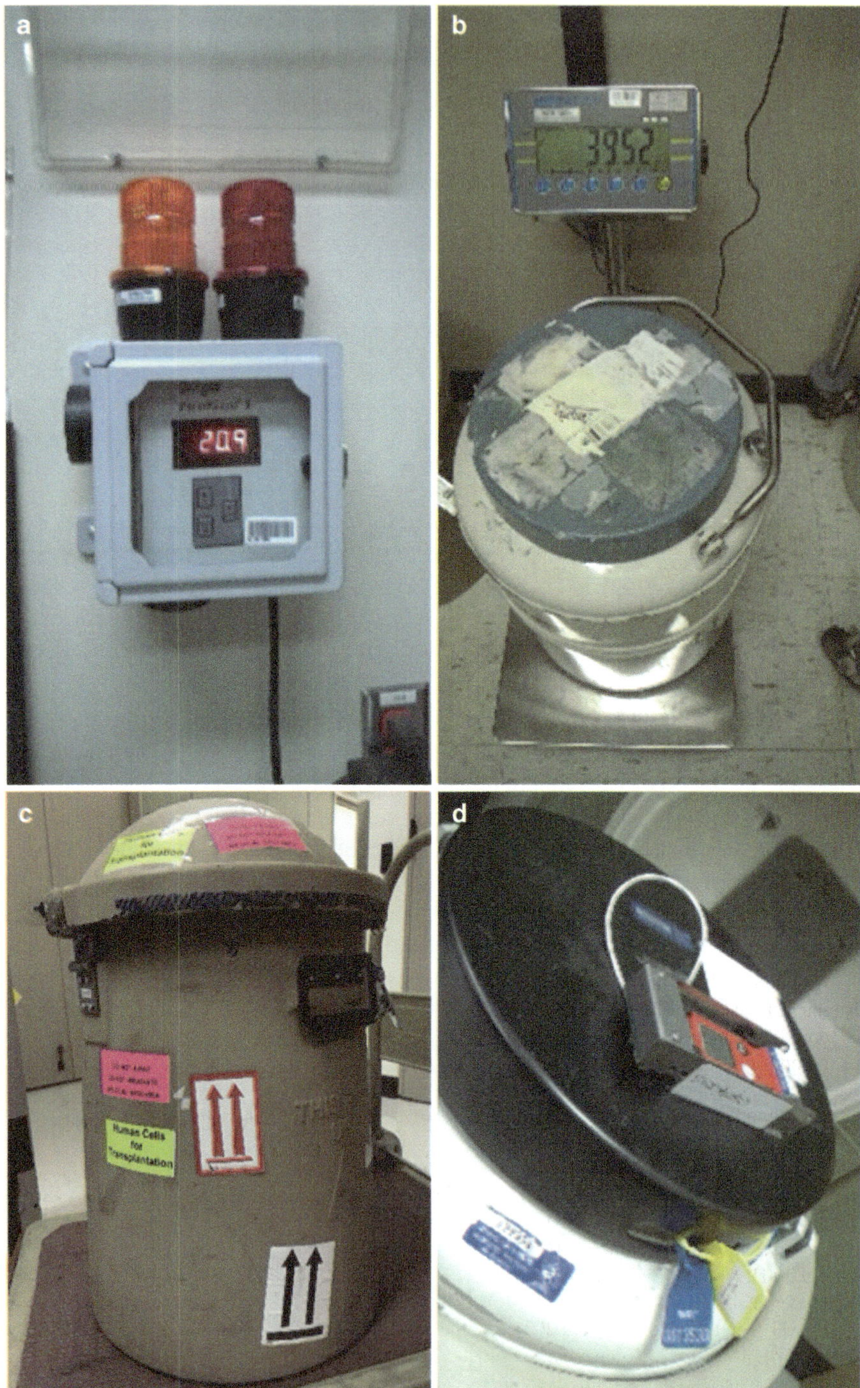

Fig. 12.4 (**a**) Oxygen level sensor, (**b**) charged dry shipper weight, (**c**) packaging and labeling, and (**d**) tamper proofing the dry shipper

Table 12.1 An example of instructions on charging a dry shipper

Time duration for certain steps will vary from one facility to another depending on the performance qualification
1. Remove the cork/cover of the vapor shipper by lifting straight up (do not twist)
2. Fill the dry shipper cavity just above the upper cavity holes but below the neck tube
3. Replace the cork/cover and allow the dry shipper to cool down for 30 min
4. Refill the dry shipper cavity according to step #2
5. Allow the dry shipper to hold the liquid N2 for 48 h
6. Pour off the remaining liquid N2, and record the weight the dry shipper
7. The dry shipper is now charged and ready for use

excess liquid N2 so that it is no longer considered as a "dangerous good" by the US Department of Transportation (DOT) or the International Air Transport Association (IATA). Dry shipper should then be packaged and labeled in accordance with applicable laws and regulations (Fig. 12.4c). An appropriate amount of absorbent packing material should also surround the packaged product to minimize physical perturbation of the enclosed product. Finally, dry shippers should be secured with tamper-proof ties (Fig. 12.4d) but should not be so tightly sealed as to allow pressure to build up within the container; otherwise, abnormal spikes in the temperature tracing may be detected as predicted by ideal gas laws.

12.5 Regulations for Packaging, Labeling, and Documentation

The procedures for the packaging and labeling of transfer containers are designed to maintain the integrity of the CT product while protecting the health and safety of personnel involved in the transfer process (The Foundation for the Accreditation of Cellular Therapy (FACT) and the Joint Accreditation Committee ISCT and EBMT 2015). It is the responsibility of the transfer facility to properly classify, package, label, and document the substance being shipped in accordance with applicable laws and regulations to allow for positive identification and to inform the courier of the appropriate handling of the biological and cryogenic material (AABB 2015). For CT products transferring on public roads, the outer container should be affixed with at least the following labels (if applicable) (The Foundation for the Accreditation of Cellular Therapy (FACT) and the Joint Accreditation Committee ISCT and EBMT 2015):

- Statement of "Do Not X-Ray" and/or "Do Not Irradiate"
- Statements of "Human Cells for Administration" or equivalent and "Handle with Care"
- Shipper handling instructions
- Transfer facility name, street address, contact person, and phone number
- Receiving facility name, street address, contact person, and phone number

For domestic interstate transfer by ground or air, the US DOT regulations for the proper packaging and labeling for each hazard category apply. When CT products are transferred internationally, most air carriers adopt the IATA Dangerous Goods Regulations and the Technical Instructions of the ICAO. The IATA defines "dangerous goods" as "articles or substances which are capable of posing a significant risk to the health, safety, property, or the environment." Both the IATA and ICAO adopt the recommendations of the United Nations Committee of Experts on the Transport of Dangerous Goods for the international transport of infectious substances and clinical specimens.

12.5.1 Dry Shippers Are Considered a Non-dangerous Good

The US DOT has determined that the use of liquid N2 charged dry shippers fall within the regulatory exceptions for "atmospheric gases" provided in Title 49 of the Code of Federal Regulations (Code of Federal Regulations n.d.). Airlines allow the transfer of dry shippers in accordance with the IATA Dangerous Goods Regulations 2.3.A—"Insulated packaging containing refrigerated liquid N2 (dry shipper) fully absorbed in a porous material containing only non-dangerous goods." Furthermore, the ICAO technical packing instructions 202 for refrigerated liquefied gases in an open cryogenic receptacle are also applicable and must be followed.

12.5.2 Exempt Human Specimen

The regulatory requirements for *donor eligibility* determination has meant that the majority of CT products are classified as exempt human specimen with minimal likelihood of containing infectious pathogens in a form that would cause infection. However, appropriate packaging and labeling requirements must be followed to further minimize the risk of exposure (International Civil Aviation Organization (ICAO) n.d.):

- A leak-proof primary receptacle(s)
- A leak-proof secondary packaging (such as a resealable bag) with enough absorbent material to contain the contents of the product in the event of a leak
- A leak-proof outer container constructed to "withstand leakage of contents, impact shocks, pressure changes, temperature changes, puncture, and other conditions incident to ordinary handling" (The Foundation for the Accreditation of Cellular Therapy (FACT) and the Joint Accreditation Committee ISCT and EBMT 2015)

12.5.3 Biological Substance, Category B

In situations where risk factors for, and clinical evidence of, infection due to a relevant communicable disease agent or disease (RCDAD) were identified based upon the results of donor screening and testing, the CT product is classified as Biological Substance, Category B (UN 3373) with additional packaging and labeling requirements (International Air Transport Association (IATA) n.d.). RCDAD is defined by 21 CFR §1271.3(r) to include the human immunodeficiency virus 1 and virus 2, hepatitis B virus, hepatitis C virus, human transmissible spongiform encephalopathy, treponema pallidum, and human T-lymphotropic virus type I and type II. Some of the key differences from exempt human specimen include:

- Category B infectious substances must be packaged in a triple packaging consisting of a primary receptacle, a secondary packaging, and a rigid outer packaging.
- The outer container must be labeled with a "UN 3373" diamond-shaped mark adjacent to a statement of "Biological Substances, Category B."
- The packaging must be capable of successfully passing the drop test at a drop height of at least 1.2 m.
- The packaging must be capable of withstanding pressure differential of 95 kPa in the range of −40 to −55 °C.

12.6 Chain of Custody and Receipt of CT Product

At each step of the transfer process, beginning with collection and including each service where the CT product is handled all the way to the transplant/infusion center, a chain of custody document needs to accompany the product. It should have vital information on the product and be signed by the staff or service member transferring the product and the staff or service member receiving the product as well as the time the transfer took place. Commercial shipping companies have computerized scanning processes that handle their legs of transport. Either manual or electronic methods could be employed, but each product should have an unbroken record chain of where it was at any time during the process and who was responsible for it.

The timing of transferring a CT product should be mutually agreed upon by the consigner (transfer facility) and consignee (receiving facility). The courier's itinerary should be communicated in detail to the receiving facility so that trained personnel are available to document the integrity of the outer container, record the TMD status indicator, open the dry shipper, inspect the CT product for evidence of mishandling or microbial contamination, and verify the labeling and paperwork documentation (The Foundation for the Accreditation of Cellular Therapy (FACT) and the Joint Accreditation Committee ISCT and EBMT 2015). There should be complete summary records to allow the receiving facility to review and verify the CT product specification (e.g., NMDP or the package insert for FDA-approved CT products) and the allogeneic donor eligibility before making a decision to accept, reject, or quarantine the CT product. In addition to these accompanying documents, the transfer facility should also provide thawing procedures and a return airbill for the prompt return of the dry shipper for quality control and maintenance of the dry shipper inventory. For cryopreserved products, the receiving facility should transfer the CT product into a storage freezer kept at or below −150 °C before the hold time of the dry shipper elapses.

12.7 Case Study #1: Transport of Non-cryopreserved HPC, Apheresis Product

A transplant center outside of the USA requests a HPC, apheresis, product from a collection center located within the USA. The collection center informs the transplant center that a 1-day collection is planned, but the international courier booked a flight to arrive in the USA on day 2—just in case the collection goal was not achieved on day 1. The collection goal of 480 × 10^6 CD34$^+$ cells with a viability of 99% was achieved on day 1, but no courier was available. Therefore, the CT product was stored overnight in a refrigerator at 2–8 °C to minimize loss of viability.

On day 2, when the courier arrived, the primary product bag was placed in a resealable secondary container and transferred in a validated, thermally insulated container with a room temperature gel pack (specifically requested by the transplant center). Due to flight connection delays, the HPC apheresis product did not arrive at the transplant center until day 3 with a viability of 45%. The temperature tracings during transport were within acceptable limits 18–24 °C. What are the failures in this case, and what corrective and preventative actions could have been taken?

Discussion: First, there was a communication failure that resulted in the international courier arriving at the collection facility 1 day late. Second, if the collection facility was made aware of the courier's delayed itinerary during the apheresis collection procedure on day 1, then autologous plasma could have been collected and added to the CT product to improve cell viability during prolonged transfer (Leemhuis et al. 2014). Third, the optimal temperature for maintaining CD34$^+$ cell viability is at refrigerated temperature (Antonenas et al. 2006).

12.8 Case Study #2: Transfer of Cryopreserved HPC, Cord Blood Unit

A transplant center outside of the USA requests a HPC, cord blood unit (CBU) from a licensed cord blood bank in the USA. A cryopreserved CBU is packaged and shipped in a vacuum-insulated dry shipper containing vapor N2 along with an electronic data logger for continuous temperature monitoring. Regulatory requirements for the labeling and documentation of an exempt human specimen were followed. Chain of custody was clearly documented from the transfer facility to the receiving facility via a courier service. Upon receipt of and opening of the outer container of the dry shipper, the electronic data logger displayed an alarm mode. The contents of the dry shipper appear undisturbed. Examination of the temperature tracings reveals a plateau pattern followed by a tall spike. What is the likely cause of these temperature deviations, and are these temperature deviations likely to be harmful to the cryopreserved CBU product?

Discussion: An investigation revealed that the timing of the 4.5-h temperature plateau coincided exactly with the flight itinerary. A buildup of pressure within the dry shipper container would explain the observed temperature deviation as predicted by ideal gas laws. Then 8 h after the airplane lands, the transplant center opened and closed the dry shipper. The post-thaw viability of the cryopreserved CBU product was acceptable and the recipient engrafted within the expected time frame. To prevent pressure buildup within the dry shipper, the cork lid of the dry shipper should be positioned to allow venting of vapor N2, and the tamper-proof ties should be secure but not be excessively tightened.

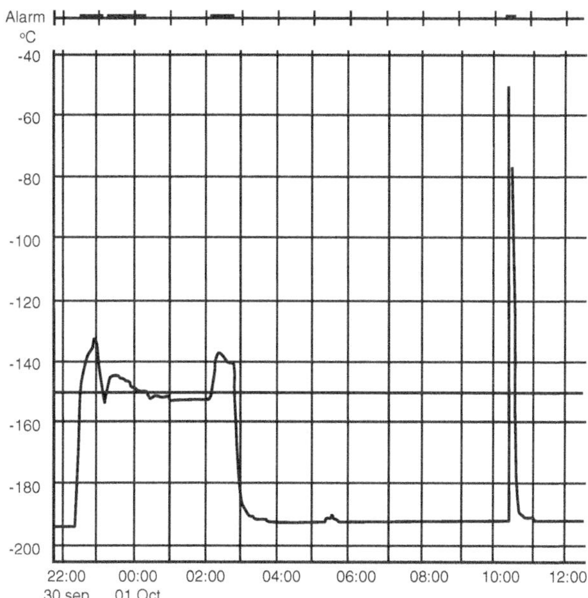

References

AABB (2015) Standards for cellular therapy services, 7th edn. AABB Publications, Bethesda, MD

Antonenas V, Garvin F, Webb M et al (2006) Fresh PBSC harvests, but not BM, show temperature-related loss of CD34 viability during storage and transport. Cytotherapy 8:158–165

Code of Federal Regulations (n.d.) Title 49 CFR—Transportation—Parts 171–180—hazardous materials regulations

Donaldson C, Armitage WJ, Denning-Kendall PA et al (1996) Optimal cryopreservation of human umbilical cord blood. Bone Marrow Transplant 18:725–731

International Air Transport Association (IATA) (n.d.). Dangerous Goods Regulations 2.3A. Packing instructions 650

International Civil Aviation Organization (ICAO) (n.d.) Technical instructions for the safe transport of dangerous goods by air. Packing instructions 202

Leemhuis T, Padley D, Keever-Taylor C et al (2014) Essential requirements for setting up a stem cell processing laboratory. Bone Marrow Transplant 49:1098–1105

Olson WC, Smolkin ME, Farris EM et al (2011) Shipping blood to a central laboratory in multicenter clinical trials: effect of ambient temperature on specimen temperature, and effects of temperature on mononuclear cell yield, viability, and immunologic function. J Transl Med 9:26

The Foundation for the Accreditation of Cellular Therapy (FACT) and the Joint Accreditation Committee ISCT and EBMT (2015) International standards for hematopoietic cellular therapy collection, processing, and administration, 6th edn. http://www.jacie.org/standards/6th-edition-2015. Accessed 10 Jan 2017

Wada RK, Bradford A, Moogk M et al (2004) Cord blood units collected at a remote site: a collaborative endeavor to collect umbilical cord blood through the Hawaii Cord Blood Bank and store the units at the Puget Sound Blood Center. Transfusion 44:111–118

Yang H, Acker JP, Hannon J et al (2011) Damage and protection of UC blood cells during cryopreservation. Cytotherapy 3:377–386

GPSR Compliance

The European Union's (EU) General Product Safety Regulation (GPSR) is a set of rules that requires consumer products to be safe and our obligations to ensure this.

If you have any concerns about our products, you can contact us on ProductSafety@springernature.com

In case Publisher is established outside the EU, the EU authorized representative is:

Springer Nature Customer Service Center GmbH
Europaplatz 3
69115 Heidelberg, Germany

Batch number: 09640703

Printed by Printforce, the Netherlands